Zika Virus

The Pregnancy Plague

Richard Mertens

DEDICATION

For Librarians.
Organizing knowledge so we can
reference the world.

ACKNOWLEDGMENTS

The mosquito. Otherwise we'd obsess about the cockroach.

Contents

Red Flag

"Everybody has a plan until they get punched in the mouth" --Mike Tyson, boxer.

In 1947, researchers working in the Uganda Zika forest discovered the Zika virus while gathering data on yellow fever and its presence in wildlife. The virus appeared harmless enough even though the vector for the Zika virus, the mosquito, specifically the *Aedes aegypti*, was a known disease vector for attention grabbing conditions such as malaria, yellow fever, West Nile and dengue.

Researchers gave it little more thought, relegating it to some obscure corner of medical academia where it languished. No one observed any noticeable medical condition associated with the Zika virus other than a couple of cases of mild flu like symptoms, so there was no concern. Besides, the *Aedes aegypti* mosquito had an affinity more for monkeys than it did people. In urban areas, *A. aegypti* fared poorly compared to how well it flourished on the rural northern shores of Lake Victoria of Uganda's southern border. Even Ugandans had no knowledge of the Zika virus until very recently, likely due to the same African human population resistance that also provides some protection against more serious diseases of dengue, yellow fever and West Nile.

70 years later, the Zika virus has exploded into our awareness from South America's Brazil, home to the 2016 summer Olympics. Brazil's one piece of good news was the anticipated arrival of the world's nations for the largest recurring sports spectacle on earth. However, even the grandiosity of the summer Olympics has not been enough to save it from a multitude of embarrassments, namely an ongoing unraveling political scandal involving the state owned oil company Petrobas, going all the way up to the office of the president. Additionally, the Olympic water venues for triathletes and boating events have been found to be essentially toxic raw sewage after a 5 month long Associated Press investigation discovered the sailing event venues loaded with rotavirus, enterovirus and fecal coliforms. The concentrations were determined to be significant enough that only three teaspoons of water would be enough to make a person sick. One potential South Korean Olympian wind sailed a water venue and became so sick he needed to be hospitalized for nearly a week. This discovery was made no less than at one of Brazil's most famous beaches, the Copacabana beach where thousands of tourists are expected to try to enjoy the water. (Associated Press 2015)[1] Literally, swimming in your own toilet would be more hygienic because at least you would be exposed to your own family's biome and not an entire city's viral and bacterial slough.

So Brazil's ambitious coming out party, with the Olympics being sort of a world bar mitzvah to celebrate its arrival as a major presence in the global economy, is losing its glow in the shadows of corruption and pollution. As if that weren't enough to disappoint Brazilians, news has arrived that hundreds of monstrous looking babies are being born with malformed heads, i.e. microcephaly.

In October 2015, Brazil's Ministry of Health reported a notable uptick in the number of cases of microcephaly in the northeast state of Pernambuco. The normal rate for the state of Pernambuco came in at about 10 cases of microcephaly annually. The first 11 months of 2015 tallied 141 cases of microcephaly in 44 of Pernambuco's 185 municipalities.[2].

Clusters happen. In the broadest sense, epidemiology is the science of tracking characteristics. For most of us, we hear the word 'epidemiology' and likely start thinking of investigations of where a disease outbreak began. That is accurate. However, epidemiologists do not merely track the abnormal in the negative sense but the abnormal positive as well, whatever the measure may be. Many epidemiologists are just as curious as to why certain populations or epochs of time display a notable quality such as longevity or high IQ as they are about the 2015 Chipotle restaurant chain *e. coli* origins. They want to get to the source of the cause that makes a trait more pronounced than normal in the general population.

But what's abnormal? After observing a series of events, we can began to predict how often something should happen. Flip a coin a few thousand times and you'll soon observe that it works out to be that half of the flips will yield heads and the other half tails. You will also notice there will be streaks of 3, 4, 5 flips in a row of one or the other and other patterns. If you flipped a quarter five times where it all came up heads, that would be a rough approximation of a cluster in medicine, or about a 3% chance or as odds of 33:1. The odds of flipping 5 heads in a row are roughly 1 out of 33 series of 5 flip sets. Also, abnormal is often defined as outside the parameters of two standard deviations where the first deviation is 34% either side of the median on a standard distribution curve and the second deviation is about 13% either side beyond the 34% of the median. It looks like this:

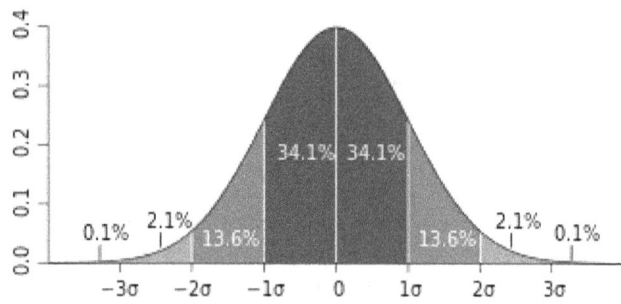

(Wikipedia 2016)[3]

In Pernambuco enough cases of microcephaly have occurred out of the range of normal, or two standard deviations, that it is considered a cluster.

Do not let the above illustration lead you to believe that microcephaly happens 1 out of 33 times or 3% of the time. It doesn't. The normal occurrence of such is about 10 times a year per 129,000 births in the state of Pernambuco according to 2014 Brazil Ministry of Health records. When the rate of such cases jumps to 141 per year that's well outside of the two standard deviations of normal occurrence and attracts the label of cluster since it happened in a defined geographic area.

Clusters are red flags. Doctors began reporting their findings to the Brazil Ministry of Health which in turn informed the Pan American Health Organization and World Health Organization.

Soon the states of Rio Grande do Norte and Paraiba reported increases of births of microcephalic infants between August and November of 2015. This prompted Brazil's Ministry of Health to issue an alert 17 November 2015 via PAHO and WHO to member States. Reading the alert document, one could easily be lulled into the sense that the observed increases are more of a routine caution than a flashing warning. (Pan American Health

Organization/World Health Organization 2015)[4]

In November 2015, the medical community in Brazil started having a red flag waved in its face. To their credit, Brazil MOH watched and investigated, their observations backed up with blood tests and ultra sounds of pregnant women.

If you read the PAHO/WHO alert issued back in November 2015, you will notice in the sidebar notes general causes of microcephaly are genetic abnormalities and environmental factors. No mention of the Zika virus is made. However, the blood tests eventually began to show a very high correlation between mothers testing positive for Zika also giving birth to microcephalic babies. Although health officials stress strongly that they cannot show a direct cause and effect of microcephaly being caused by the Zika virus, the numbers are too compelling to dismiss it and thus we reasonably conclude there is indeed a cause and effect occurring.

The next red flag that has appeared is the sudden rise in Brazil of Guillain-Barre syndrome, a nerve condition that results in increasing paralysis over a period of several days. This is a particularly nasty aspect of Zika since those afflicted are dealing with a neurological disorder and diseases of the nerves are difficult to treat and carry pessimistic prognosis in terms of long term disability or death.

What happens during Guillain-Barre is that a person's own immune system attacks the myelin sheathing surrounding the nerves in a protective coating. Like the insulation you would find on an electrical wire in a typical home to protect against electrical arcing with other conductive objects, especially metal ones, myelin performs essentially the same function in making sure electrical nerve impulses remain on track to their intended destination to help you lift your arm, swallow, breathe and function in every possible way as a person. Without myelin, nerve impulses would just dissipate into your bodily fluids, useless to signal conscious and unconscious bodily functions.

As of this writing, Brazil has reported over 400 cases where victims of Guillain-Barre have tested positive for Zika. Again, health officials are insisting they cannot provide direct evidence of cause and effect between Zika and Guillain-Barre but the strong correlation between G-B victims also testing positive for Zika where the surge in cases of microcephaly have occurred may add up to more than coincidence.

Up until January 2016, the condition was so rare that Brazil's Ministry of Health did not ask health personnel to track it. But last year, hospitals and clinics in the hard hit state of Pernambuco, the state hardest hit by the Zika virus thus far, have tallied hundreds of Guillain-Barré cases, forcing physicians to raise the issue of a possible Zika connection. (Seattle Times 2016)[5]

Possible? No. Very likely is a better description and one I believe is even slightly understated. Brazil's health system is built around what it knows, what it has learned over lifetimes are the foreseeable medical needs and health concerns of most of its citizens. Today the red flags are everywhere that Brazil has a national health disaster on its hands and it is threatening to pressure them in ways they can't predict.

Panic hasn't taken hold in Brazil, at least not the screaming in the streets type of panic we saw in 2014 with the West Africa Ebola crisis where politicians couldn't resist publicly flogging the Ebola medical responders, trying portray feats of civil liberty infringements as some sort of touching concern for their constituents.

The World Health Organization and Pan America Health Organization held an emergency meeting. On 28 January 2016, WHO Director General Margaret Chan issued a special statement from Geneva expressing profound concern, hinting strongly at that time it would declare the Zika situation an international health emergency. Four days later, WHO did indeed declare Zika an international health emergency, thus allowing itself to set in motion the logistics to make sharing of information and resources more efficient and responsive.

WHO appears to be more proactive with Zika in large part due to the very recent memories and lessons of the Ebola crisis. With the Ebola crisis, critics leveled accusations that WHO was too slow and tepid in its initial response, that their inaction allowed what was a manageable issue to bloom into an international disaster.

Brazil is not alone. It is now acknowledged that Columbia is the second hardest hit nation at this writing. The latest figures from Colombia show 20,297 confirmed cases of Zika as of February 1, 2016 with 2,116 cases of microcephalic infants, backing up Chan's assessment of an international emergency. (Haroon Siddique 2016)[6]

Per the United States Center for Disease Control, as of February 1, 2016 the Zika virus has been discovered in the Caribbean islands of Barbados, Curaçao, Dominican Republic, Guadeloupe, Haiti, Jamaica, Martinique, the US territory Commonwealth of Puerto Rico, Saint Martin and the U.S. Virgin Islands. In Central America, affected countries include Costa Rica, El Salvador, Guatemala, Honduras, Mexico, Nicaragua and Panama. The South American countries of Bolivia, Brazil, Colombia, Ecuador, French Guiana, Guyana, Paraguay, Suriname and Venezuela are seeing increasing reports of Zika transmission. The Pacific Islands of American Samoa, Samoa and Tongo report several cases as well as French Polynesia. The only African nation reporting infections are Cape Verde islands.

There are three levels of travel alerts for the above named countries. The first level is marked in green and advises to take the usual precautions such as up to date vaccines and attentive hygiene. The third level is marked red and advises to avoid travel to a listed area at all costs.

The best way to think of the difference between the first and third levels is at the first level one shouldn't drink the local water while the third level is something like the hard hit Ebola countries of West Africa.

The second level of travel advisory issued by the CDC is the yellow alert level and this type of alert provides specific actions to take while in a listed yellow alert country, up to and including advising certain persons vulnerable to certain disease(s) to avoid travel to yellow alert countries.

The genie is out of the bottle regards the Zika virus and in basically about a 6 month period it is now in more than 25 countries. Zika is on the march and only a matter of time before it is in every country in the western hemisphere with only the most extreme latitudes of Canada, Chile and Argentina not likely to be affected. *A. aegypti* doesn't much care about international borders and is not adverse to hitchhiking a ride regards air or ground travel.

The tsunami of Zika is gathering momentum and the crest of the swell is far from having been reached a maximum in the northern hemisphere. The warmer spring, summer and fall months will agitate and complicate any actions taken to combat the spread of the Zika virus.

Every country and every health system has a plan on paper for how to deal with an emergency, be it natural disasters, war or disease. However, no one really gets a chance to practice real life scenarios so the learning curves are steep and littered with potential explosive errors yet undiscovered. It's going to be exactly like former boxer Mike Tyson said: "Everyone has a plan until they get punched in the mouth."

The Mosquito

No one on planet earth has ever avoided the mosquito. It is the most well known flying insect on the planet, maybe rivaled only by the house fly. But the house fly, a capable enough vector for transmitting bacteria and some viruses, in no way competes with the mosquito for the title of disease vector.

The entire family of mosquitoes is known by the classification of *Culcidae*. Within that family are over 3,500 identified kinds of mosquitoes divided into two subfamilies known as *Anophelinae* and *Culcinae* and 41 genera with Culcinae broken down into 11 categories of tribes. The United States has 172 kinds of identified mosquito. It is easy to see how such taxonomy might overwhelm even dedicated entomologists.

The mosquito in its present form seems to have been around for about the last 80 million years with one mosquito fossil having been found preserved in Canadian amber and another in Burmese amber. So the next time you swat a mosquito away from your face, be grateful and recall that the Tyrannosaurus Rex had front limbs too short to do the same. Even Jesus Christ accepted the inevitably of mosquitoes, never bothering to make them part of any sort of miraculous triumph. It was just probably easier to walk on water than to rid his world of mosquitoes.

Luckily for us, there is a well of information on the worst offenders in the mosquito world, enough so that we can identify the worst of the worst out of a buggy lineup. If there were to be a Most Wanted poster of the mosquito that troubles man the most it would be *Aedes aegypti.*

The *A. aegypti* belongs in the Anophelinae subfamily and is distributed up and down Central and South America, central-west central and southern Africa, India, southeast Asia, northeast Australia and the southern United States. It has increased its range by about three fold since the 1970's when environmental concerns over the use of widespread chemical control took hold and mosquito control efforts faded away. The current range matches the range of the 1930's before widespread control efforts took place.

A. aegypti is not the only carrier of Zika. *Aedes albopictus* has also been implicated as a carrier. *A. albopictus* is also known as the Asian Tiger mosquito and its range has steadily expanded as well. In the United States, it was initially detected at a Houston port in 1985 lurking in a shipment of used tires. From there it spread across the south and up the eastern seaboard to become established in the northeast. It was found in southern California in 2001, eliminated for a period then found again in 2013 in Los Angeles. North American habitat that suits the environmental conditions of the Asian Tiger mosquito is expected to more than triple in size in the next twenty years, especially in urban areas where the majority of populations now live. (Wikipedia 2016)[7]

The range for both types of mosquitoes has increased in large part due to increased commercial trade as products and people travel more freely across international borders, bringing with them our increased exposure to arboviruses which are any types of viruses spread by mosquitoes. Dengue, yellow fever, chikungunya and Zika are arboviruses, well known nasty tropical diseases that are painful and which sometimes leave permanent disability or death as a calling card. An example closer to home for many of us with dogs is prophylactic heart worm medicine given monthly to Rover to prevent infection by mosquitoes. The following CDC map illustrates the current distribution of both types of mosquitoes as of this writing February, 2016.

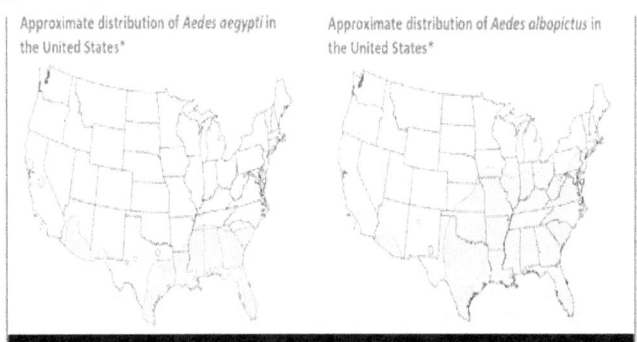

Approximate distribution of *Aedes aegypti* in the United States*

Approximate distribution of *Aedes albopictus* in the United States*

(US Dept of Health and Human Services 2016)[8]

From the maps you can see that between the *A. albopictus* and *A. aegypti* that they inhabit about a third of the United States, that area below the Mason-Dixon line and Ohio River and east of the Mississippi along with a large portion of Texas and scattered areas in Arizona and California. The one respite these areas will get from the spread of Zika are the cooler winter months when mosquito activity in general is suppressed or absent. Come the warmer months of spring and summer, it is not a guess if US residents will have to deal with Zika infection but how many will have to deal with Zika infection.

Of the 3,500 types of mosquitoes, the Asian tiger mosquito (Aedes albopictus) and the yellow fever (Aedes aegypti) mosquito are the two that are becoming the fast menace.

Both mosquitoes have similar characteristics in anatomy,

behavior and habitat needs. It is the female that is the aggressor in that it needs a blood meal in order to develop its eggs. The proboscis used to drill through skin excretes a saliva that contains an anticoagulant to facilitate the blood extraction and the common human reaction to this saliva is a redness and itching at the bite site. The female proboscis is more developed than the male proboscis and is sensitive enough to detect capillary action below the skin surface. This is why if you ever watched a mosquito on your own skin you may have noticed that she spent some time probing the area before settling in to make the lunge through your epidermis. If she isn't satisfied with the prospects, she may simply leave.

Mosquitoes engage in what is general movement and are opportunistic in their hunt for a blood meal. Carbon dioxide we exhale is widely believed to be the main trigger attractant though many experts across the literature believe that lactic acid, ammonia and octenol are as important. Octenol is also known as mushroom alcohol and it is contained in our breath and sweat. Octenol is also used in conjunction with carbon dioxide as a bait for insect traps designed to kill them. It is what is widely used as bait in the neon violet bug zappers that so many of us delight in as they crackle and snap away during the evening hours.

The typical life cycle of our two mosquitoes is that they go through four stages. The first stage is the egg stage and the females have a bobbing behavior similar to that of dragonflies and mayflies. This bobbing behavior is also known as dapping and any trout fisherman worth his $800 Orvis fly rod knows exactly the right time of the season that mayflies are out and he knows all about dapping after the big hatch.

The typical mosquito egg is oblong and has buoys to assist the eggs to float. In their lifetime females lay about 100–200 eggs in rafts on or over standing water that are about 1/8-1/4 inch in length. One mating pair can create several generations and thousands of new mosquitoes in a single season. A typical lifespan of an adult *A. aegypti* is 15 to 30 days depending on habitat and weather, the eggs can survive for as long as a year in a dry state, thus allowing the mosquitoes to re-emerge after surviving the winter months or drought.

Once the eggs hatch in the water upon which they were dropped, they are known as larva. These tiny little larva use a breathing tube called a trumpet that functions pretty much like a snorkeling tube, so they must come to the surface frequently to catch their breath. When they aren't breathing they are feeding on single cell life of bacteria, algae and other minute organisms appropriate to their own size. As larva, they molt several times by shedding an outer shell and grow further. After several molts they achieve a size that can be discerned by our own eyes. If you ever had a kiddy swimming pool in your backyard and left the water unchanged for a period of several weeks, you've no doubt looked into it and wondered what those little 'minnows' were and how they got there. They aren't at all fish but mosquito larva and pupa.

The third stage is the pupa stage and here at this stage they just basically hangout by floating just below the surface of the water, their breathing tube holding them up. If annoyed by a passerby, they will disperse from below the surface and squiggle into deeper water. After a couple of days of this existence they bob up to the surface where their backside splits and out comes a shiny new mosquito with a mission in life to make more mosquitoes.

The adult stage is the fourth stage. If conditions are just so the mosquito can develop from egg to adult in as little as 4 to 6 days but the normal is considered to be around 40 days. Adult mosquitoes usually mate within a few days after emerging from the pupal stage. In most species, the males demonstrate swarming behavior, especially around the dusk and dawn hours. The females crash into these swarms to mate and fertilize their eggs.

Males typically live for about 5 to 7 days, finding sources of nourishment with nectar and other sources of sugar. After loading up on a protein rich blood meal, females rest for several days as the blood supper is digested and eggs form. This all depends on the weather, but usually takes only 2 to 3 days in warm and humid conditions. When the eggs are fully developed, the female drops the eggs while dapping and begins her hunt anew for a new victim from which to extract a blood meal.

The cycle repeats itself until the female dies, which is only about 14 days in the wild. They can live longer if they manage to avoid predators and if weather conditions are conducive to an extended life span. The single largest factor is the ability to obtain a blood meal.

Getting around, locomotion, is fairly impressive considering the typical mosquito is only about a third of an inch long. They can reach speeds of up to 10 mph and are not adverse to riding a breeze, though they tend to cling to a solid object in high winds. It has been observed that a mosquito can travel up to 8 to 10 miles in day.

Humans are a natural target but pretty much any mammal is a target. Heavy breathers and people or animals who generate a lot of body heat are targets since mosquitoes have heat sensing abilities. It isn't your imagination to conclude that performing active outdoor physical labor attracts swarms of mosquitoes to yourself. The average mosquito has 72 smelling sensors on its antennae and 27 of those are honed in on smells specific to human sweat. (Devlin 2010)[9]

Mosquitoes can be found on every single place on the planet except maybe Iceland and Antarctica. Mosquito larva have been observed in Iceland but the peculiar weather patterns of mid winter thaws and freezes appear to kill off any emerging populations.

If cold weather halts mosquitoes in Iceland and

Antarctica, then why are places like Alaska, Minnesota and Canada thick every summer with swarms? It is the pupa and larva that are vulnerable to the cold weather. Adults are able to endure freezing temperature thanks to a sort of antifreeze that kicks in when the days become shorter and temperatures began to drop. This is referred to as diapause, a sort of hibernation. Diapause is triggered by shortening daylight in combination with temperature drops. Contrary to popular belief, a frosty fall night does not kill off the adult mosquitoes but merely appears to physiologically trigger them, in combination with the shorter periods of daylight, to become inactive. And like a bear will gorge itself prior to its hibernation, mosquitoes in temperate areas appear to become more active in securing fats, proteins and sugars. The three sources of nutrition provide sustenance for a very slowed metabolism, a food store to draw upon when awakening and protection from drying out that comes with low humidity conditions during the winter months.

Eggs also survive the winter months and when the temperature and humidity reaches a certain point, the eggs will develop and hatch.

We know there are over 3,500 kinds of mosquitoes and not all them behave identically regards the weather and environment. What has made the *A. aegypti* and *A. albopictus* so well known amongst those who need to know about mosquitoes is both have displayed a strong ability to adapt from more rural environments to more urban environments where the average residential area provides shelter, food and places to breed.

Standing pools of water such as mud puddles and swampy low areas are the types of areas we often associate with suitable mosquito egg laying. However, urbanization has created all sorts of containers where water may sit undisturbed for days or weeks at a time. A drive through the average suburb will reveal that we have built ponds to catch rainy run off, built beautiful parks and golf courses that are watered consistently through dry periods and watered enough that any standing water is replenished before it evaporates. While agriculture and other land use drained swampy mosquito habitat in the more rural areas, our urbanization has reduced the impact of these actions on the mosquito reproductive cycle.

The average home has about 50 meters (164 feet) of rain gutter along the roofline. Any person who has ever risked their very neck to teeter on a ladder to clean gutters to enable uninterrupted flow knows that there is often standing water. This is a near perfect environment where eggs, larvae and pupae are sheltered from predators and drying winds. The largest risk is more water, read rain, that fills gutters enough to wash away eggs, pupae and larvae down to a place that can dry out, killing larva and pupae.

Golf course ponds, roadside ditches, water gardens and bird baths are other near ideal egg laying environments for mosquitoes. There is an additional boost from these types of standing waters and that is they are usually shallow, meaning they can be warmed quickly and retain enough heat over brief cooling periods that they become near ideal mosquito egg incubators, hastening the first three stages of the life cycle and, in turn, hastening the creation of successive generations that will swarm your evening barbeque.

The mosquito's imposition upon the collective human conscience is due to its global presence and presence in large numbers. It seems we are never dealing with just one mosquito but swarms of tens or hundreds or even thousands. What it lacks in physical attributes it overcomes with sheer numbers, the likely global population topping out at over a trillion. With a number that large it is easy to comprehend how even 0.1 of 1% of mosquitoes can be a serious health risk to humans, livestock, birds and other animals. It is no accident that much of medicine is predicated upon us reacting to mosquito borne diseases in efforts to reduce the severity and risk to the global population. Soon enough we will see exactly how we react to a mosquito threat.

The Zika Virus

A virus is much smaller than a bacteria. Bacteria can be studied under more traditional glass eye piece microscopes, large enough to be subject to magnification and observed under the right conditions of light, stain and slide preparation. Bacteria are single cell organisms that contain a cell membrane and a nuclei but most distinctively are able to multiply on their own under the right conditions and, by way of contrast and comparison, help us understand viruses.

There are three domains of cellular life:

Domain Eukaryotes include fungi, plants and animals and pretty much comprise the life forms we interact with on a daily level.

Domain Archaea is the oldest domain. Some examples of archaeal type organisms would be those which produce methane (swamp) gas, and extremophiles that thrive in high salt, sulfur or heat conditions or highly acidic conditions such as Yellowstone Park's famous geysers, thermal pools and mud pots. These are some of the oldest organisms on earth, likely having been with us since the earth's infancy.

Domain Bacteria contains most of the known disease

pathogens we deal with and are partially identified as either gram negative or gram positive, a method using violet stain to differentiate between the two. Common examples of gram positive bacteria would be the Staphylococcus often simply referred to as staph. MRSA, methycillin resistant staphylococcus aureus, is a gram positive bacteria we've all heard about as being a nagging problem in our hospitals. If you ever had strep throat, it was a gram positive Streptococcus bacteria. A gram negative bacteria, one that doesn't hold the violet stain when treated, would include things like E. coli and salmonella, two types of bacteria we often hear about involving food product recalls and can be lethal if not treated promptly with antibiotics.

Viruses fit into none of the above domains and cannot be observed with traditional glass magnifying microscopes, requiring electron microscopy. Real atom stuff. Unlike cellular organisms like bacteria which have a ribosome, a minute particle composed of protein and RNA (ribonucleic acid)and serves as the site for protein production encased in a fatty cellular wall, viruses have no ribosome or cell wall but instead are usually coated in a protein shell. Size wise, a virus hangs around the 20/1,000,000,000 of a meter in size while a typical red blood cell is about 5,000 billionths of a meter. Scale wise, that's about comparable to one person in a typical high school 6 lane 25 yard swimming pool.

Bacteria reproduction is asexual, a process called mitosis if you recall your high school biology. Meiosis is the other reproductive process, the process of two different cells coming together through sexual reproduction and a mixing of chromosomes contributed by an egg and a sperm to create a different entity. (Mom, Dad, you). Mitosis produces an exact replica of a cell through a four stage process of division and there is no genetic mixing like there is in meiosis, the process that made me and you.

Viruses, like bacteria, self replicate. We know that certain bacteria and other cells self replicate through mitosis, the process that is responsible for our general growth and repairs such as wound healing. While bacterial and other cells are considered alive, viruses present no clear answer as to whether they are alive or not alive. Obviously, self replication is not a sole criteria for determining if something is alive. This is a debate that may well be better suited for philosophers than it is for scientists, and if you would like to have a little fun if you ever find yourself in a group of scientists or doctors, throw out the question whether or not a virus is a living entity. I think it is a bit like Artificial Intelligence where machines build each other.

Bacteria and other self replicating cells reproduce through self division, fission. Viruses reproduce by invading a host cell, and in taking over a cell, forces the cell to make copies of the virus's own DNA or RNA. During this act of piracy, the virus often destroys the host cell, releasing the newly manufactured viruses that go on to find another host cell and continue the process.

Medically, both a virus and bacteria can be infectious but bacteria tend to be localized in infections such as you might see with an inflamed, reddish or purulent wound. By contrast, viral infections are systemic, throughout the whole of a body or plant. Further, bacteria are often beneficial such as those found in soils to aid in plant nutrition uptake or thriving in the gut to aid digestion.

Bacterial infections can be treated with antibiotics with certain antibiotics targeted to specific bacteria. Often times, various bacteria are simply narrowed down to being gram positive or gram negative and an antibiotic prescribed on that basis alone. Gram positive bacteria like staphylococci or streptococci are susceptible to penicillin, though resistance is becoming more noticeable and worrisome. Gram-negative bacteria such as E. coli and salmonella are resistant to multiple drugs and are increasingly resistant to most available antibiotics. When a bacterial infection sample is collected it is cultured in a medium called agar, a jelly-like substance derived from algae and laced with a nutrient like blood or other tissue, then observed to see which antibiotic disc placed in the culture Petri dish inhibits or destroys the bacteria in question.

Viral infections cannot be treated with antibiotics. Gram-negative bacteria are resistant to multiple drugs and are increasingly resistant to most available antibiotics. Despite persistence warnings from the US Food and Drug Administration, Centers for Disease Control and National Institutes of Health, doctors often fail to culture their patients to differentiate the virally infected from the bacterially infected and simply write out an antibiotic prescription to assuage the patient they are 'doing something'. Viruses, however, once creating an infectious state within its host, are not generally treatable with drugs in the way antibiotics work. Most treatments involved with viruses are geared towards the symptoms such as ameliorating the runny nose, muscle aches or fever. Some anti viral medications such as acyclovir for active herpes or chicken pox attempt to inhibit or interrupt the DNA replication process of a virus. Success is often mixed.

The single most effective treatment for viral infections has been prophylactic medicine, that is the use of preventive measures, namely the vaccine. Getting our shots is a part of growing up for most everyone. Common vaccinations today are for mumps, measles, rubella (MMR), chicken pox (varicella), annual influenza vaccine, pneumococcal vaccine, DTap and Tdap which contain diptheria, tetanus, and pertussis vaccine. Other common vaccines are for Hepatitis A and B, rabies and yellow fever depending on a person's employment or region of residence. Last, the one that started it all on a scale with which we are familiar, the polio vaccine developed by Jonas Salk, though I'd be remiss not mention Edward Jenner's refinement of the small pox vaccine, earning him the title of Father of Immunology.

I used information on bacteria to help understand what a virus is and isn't. We know bacteria are living organisms and aren't quite so sure if viruses are or not. We know bacteria can asexually reproduce through fission and create identical replicas of itself whereas viruses must hijack a cell and force it to manufacture more virus. Thanks to the average virus being 1/500 the size of the average bacterium, the viral invasion process is made that much easier.

Like bacteria, viruses can be moved from one plant or animal to another by a variety of means. Water is a common reservoir for many forms of bacteria and viruses so it's paramount that much of infection control focuses on water system hygiene. Think the town pump in 19th century Soho district of London and cholera. Plants and animals alike can harbor virus as well as insects so that when a vector like *A. aegypti* or *A. albopictus* feeds off the nectar or blood of its target, it becomes a reservoir, a flying mode of transmission known as a vector.

Other modes of transmission for certain viruses may require direct or indirect contact. The common influenza viruses are generally transmissible by way of touch with infected animate or inanimate subjects or by aerosolization such as with a cough or sneeze. The influenza virus, however, cannot be transmitted by mosquito since the physiology of the mosquito is not a suitable habitat for a flu virus to survive/stay intact, depending on whether or not you've decided virus are alive or not. Another mode of transmission is the fecal-oral route and, yes, it as gross as it sounds and as accurate. The Norvovirus (Norwalk virus), or winter vomiting bug, is transmitted by the fecal-oral route. For some reason, it seems to garner headlines via outbreaks on cruise ships though it certainly is as infectious on land as it is at sea.

Much to our chagrin, the mosquito is more than a suitable carrier for dengue, Chikungunya and yellow fever viruses, diseases that are spread horizontally, meaning insect to man. It is also known that the three aforementioned diseases are also transmitted vertically, meaning one mosquito can transmit the virus to another by contact such as in breeding or saliva exchanges, complicating efforts of control, forcing us to consider not merely using vaccines to stave off life threatening illness but that we must also control the mosquito itself. Why? Sadly, many people for various reasons cannot receive some vaccines due to allergies to the substance in a vaccine itself (egg product/byproduct being one such allergy trigger), health status, such as being immunocompromised by conditions as diverse as cancer or a myriad of other diseases, and availability or affordability. The shingles vaccine, such as Merck's blockbuster brand name drug Zostavax, costs about $220. (CostHelper.com 2015)[10]

With this general knowledge of bacterial and viral infectious agents, how does the Zika virus stack up? We know Zika is an arbovirus, meaning it can be transmitted by mosquito, namely *A. aegypti* and *A. albopictus* which are also vectors for other flaviviruses such as Dengue, yellow fever and West Nile. Together, these four viruses can accumulate a high enough concentration, known as a titer, to reinfect a mosquito that takes a blood meal from a person or other animal. However, a new complication has arisen regards transmission of Zika, specifically that it appears it can be sexually transmitted. A case in Dallas prompted health officials in early February, 2016 to report "…that a local resident was infected with the Zika virus by having sex with a person who had contracted the disease while traveling in Venezuela." (Washington Post 2016)[11]

Sexual transmission would seem to indicate that transmission is not merely zoonotic, animal to man, and horizontal, one species to another, but person to person just as hepatitis or HIV may be spread. This also strongly suggests that Zika may be spread through use of blood transfusions, plasma transfusions and certain organ transplants. As of early February, 2016, Brazil has reported two known cases of Zika infection via blood transfusion. (Wall Street Journal 2016)[12] As of this publication, no other modes of transmission for Zika are known and the upside is that with enough already to be concerned about, we do not need to worry about transmission by casual contact or an airborne route.

As we know, viruses take over the machinery of living cells and use the cell for its own purpose of replication. We can often get strong clues what types of cells a virus prefers by the signs and symptoms presented. For instance, with a flavivirus like dengue, we know that skin cells are vulnerable and we see the damage done through the expression of a rash. The typical systemic, whole body reaction is a fever, a sign that the body's immune system has kicked into gear with the production of antibodies to combat the invading virus.

Flaviviruses also appear to target the kidneys, testes, intestine and eyes. Infection of the intestine is expressed by the infected victim vomitting and dealing with nausea while infection of they eyes shows itself as eye redness resembling pink eye. In very serious cases many sorts of viral infections may cause encephalitis, an inflammation of brain cells that may lead to seizures or cranial pressure incompatible with life. Zika is suspected to have the ability to cause encephalitis.

How the Zika virus manages to target various cells depends on the chemical signals it reads from specific types of cells. Once the virus is satisfied it is knocking on the right doors, admission into the host cell is achieved by the virus by placement of the virus's protein case onto a host cell's receptors. The conjoined protein encased virus and cell receptor undertake endocytosis, the taking in of matter by a living cell by the process of a folding of its membrane to form a vacuole. Now that the invader has tricked a cell into allowing it entry, replication takes place by using the positive stranded RNA virus replication model, a process that is incredibly involved and too much to explain here. Suffice it to say, this viral replication process uses the machinery of the host cell to make multiple copies itself. Since the virus has no moral or ethical compunction about taking over a cell, it really has no concern about any damage it does to the host cell, either.

We know Zika has an affinity for nerve cells as well, now that cases of Guillain-Barre and microcephaly have been documented in large enough numbers that WHO has issued a call to arms, only the fourth such call it has made. This WHO declaration represents its highest level of alert and is only invoked in response to the most dire threats. 2009 was the first during the H1N1 influenza outbreak that is documented to have sickened up to 200 million across the globe; May 2014 was the second declaration when a paralyzing type of polio reappeared in Pakistan and Syria; the Ebola outbreak in West Africa was the third declaration of an international health emergency and WHO still has fresh in its memory the criticism that it was too slow to respond. (Washington Post 2016)[13]

Neurological disorders such as through birth defects or as an acute or chronic manifestation in children and adults are feared for the havoc they wreak up a person's overall ability to function physically and mentally. In many cases where neurological damage is extensive, the victim is so disabled that they are unable to comprehend the world in which they exist, engage it in any meaningful way and are often times at least partially dependent on others for basic needs and sometimes institutionally dependent for all their needs in more severe cases.

Typical physical symptoms associated with Zika occur in only in 1 of 4 or 5 infected persons. Right off the bat, the majority of people infected with Zika will never know they are infected. And that's OK as long as you aren't immunocompromised in some manner be it by chronic condition or age. After the initial infection event, in 2-7 days the symptoms that usually manifest in the unlucky 1 of 4 are headache, joint pain and conjunctivitis (pink eye) and maybe a fever, all indications your immune system has kicked into high drive and is developing antibodies to keep the virus out of your cells. This discomfort may last from a couple of days to up to two weeks. There is little you can do and the only treatment options are for the discomforts of pain and fever, meaning over the counter acetaminophen (Tylenol) to help out.

At the current time there is no vaccine and likely will not be a mass produced vaccine for at least several years. While we've had great success with vaccines against polio, rubella, diptheria and other nearly forgotten diseases, there are many other viruses that we are only moderately successful with, namely influenza which is hit and miss year to year. As for the human immunodeficiency virus, HIV, there is no vaccine despite very serious and intensive efforts to come up with even a coin flip of a chance of protection.

The good news is that for the 3 out of 4 of us who never know we have been subjected to a Zika infection, we'll develop antibodies that will protect us against a future infectious event where we might not be in such great shape to handle it, like say when we are over 80 years old or unfortunately maybe dealing with chemotherapy to beat back a diagnosed cancer of one sort or another.

The bad news is that the virus will sicken 1 of 4 it infects. In that group, the majority will tough it out, maybe miss a day or two of work and just get through and over it, inoculated against future Zika events thanks to those wonderful antibodies now present in abundance. However, within that group of 1 out 4 with symptoms, some will experience serious illness that may be evolve into chronic conditions such as orthalgia (joint pain) or parathesias (nerve pain, discomfort, numbness, tingling).

The aforementioned is written with a relatively healthy adult in mind. As I mentioned, those who are immunocompromised in some way by a chronic condition such as diabetes, HIV, cancer or age are most at risk for serious problems. I offered old age as being one reason a person may not have an up to snuff immune system but being very young can also be problematic. Most children under the age of 2 months have immune systems that are still far from vigorous but after age 1 year, young immune systems by most accounts develop fairly rapidly to deal with the majority of infectious assaults. It is no accident that many vaccines are postponed until the third month of life. Even then, most vaccines are given in low dose injections over a course of two or more times over several months. The only exception to this delay in the infant shot schedule is the Hepatitis B shot where the series of 3 shots are started at birth and given 6 months apart. Otherwise, vaccines for whooping cough, polio, diptheria, mumps, measles, rubella, chickenpox and rotavirus are delayed until at least the start of the third month until the immune system can respond properly to develop the necessary antibodies to ensure a lifetime of immunity. (Centers for Disease Control & Prevention 2016)[14]

The fear of Zika and the reason it has been declared a global health emergency is the Zika virus has shown an affinity for invading neurological cells. Neurological cells are, of course, what makes the brain function in such a manner in man as that it can even contemplate itself and is the seat of all that we are socially, emotionally and physically. Beyond the brain, there is the spinal cord, all the peripheral nerves and sensory nerves of sight, touch, smell, sound and taste. Voluntary (somatic) nerve pathways are responsible for conscious movement of locomotion and fine motor control while the autonomic (involuntary) nervous system supports breathing, circulatory systems, gastro-intestinal function and all other organ functions.

33

Not every nerve cell is the same, thus some are more prone to havoc from Zika than others. This is where Guillain-Barre, the disease of the nerves that causes paralysis in its sufferers, becomes such a concern. Also, the Zika virus has demonstrated an affinity for young, developing cerebral nerves of the fetus, damaging the nerves so extensively that fetal brain development is arrested and prospects for normal development never severely diminished, resulting in a brain half the size of normal. A simple way to illustrate how serious this is, is to simply imagine what would happen if your IQ were suddenly cut in half. Of course, a brain half its normal size no longer needs the normal sized cranial vault, thus the disturbingly small heads of those born with microcephaly.

This is where concern about Zika needs to be serious. The implications for immune naïve populations, such as in the United States, holds immense potential for economic disruption of the health systems, social services and families. Unlike a disease like Ebola where a resolution resulted in either survival or death within several weeks, Zika can leave the afflicted disabled and dependent for decades. G-B and microcephaly almost always exact a very high price from its victims and if Brazil is any indication of what we are facing in the United States, we're going to learn more about the two aforementioned conditions than most of us ever wanted to know. If you find the prospect of having to deal with a possible fever, joint pain, maybe conjunctivitis and days off from work worrisome, you should be terrified that there is the prospect of contracting Guillain-Barre or having a prospective mother dealing with a pregnancy that involves an anencephalic child.

Guillain-Barre

We somewhat covered what Guillain-Barre syndrome involves in that it is a condition of the nervous system. As you might suspect, the disease is named after the French discovers Georges Guillain and Jean Alexandre along with Andre Strohl in 1916. You may recognize that this was also the time that Europe, including France, was in the depths of World War I. All three doctors were an active part of the war effort which recruited them to serve and care for the soldiers. It was during their service the doctors observed in two soldiers the presentation of signs and symptoms of the syndrome that now bares two of the three discovers names. (Andre Strohl 2016)[15]

At this point in time, no scientist, medical institution or research group has been able to pin point any causative link between Zika and Guillain-Barre. So, what's the worry?

The worry is based on corresponding numbers. As Zika

has spread throughout South and Central America, there has been a corresponding rise in Guillain-Barre cases in those same places. Already the internet is exploding with conspiracy theories and misinformed (a nice word for 'stupid') crank 'theories' of pharmaceutical cartels unleashing bioengineered Zika in order to clean up on some sort of drug marketing scheme. While the pharmaceutical industry deserves a certain amount of suspicion and condemnation for some of their business practices, especially as regards licensing arrangements that effectively monopolize certain pharmaceutical products so they can manipulate supply in order to rationalize gross mark ups, they've never been caught introducing a disease causing agent into the population as part of a plot to market a future drug issue. That would involve them planting the virus in Uganda in 1947 and getting it to Brazil in 2015. Anyone who could come to me with that sort of investment or venture capital plan would be chalked up into the Bernie Madoff category of money management.

Nut jobs aside, there is a very real and documented observation that Guillain-Barre is increasing in prevalence in conjunction with increases in documented cases of Zika infections. How or what the pathway is from becoming Zika infected to Guillain-Barre cannot be mapped and pinpointed directly, with many clinicians and researchers leaving wiggle room to avoid making a proclamation that there is a definite link. WHO is pulling its punches as well on the link between G-B and Zika but it is also hedging their bets heavily by circulating the observed correlation between the two.

What we do understand is that a person's immune system begins to attack the body itself, creating what is called an autoimmune disease. Immune cells normally only attack virus and bacteria cells and other invading organisms they recognize as not being from the neighborhood. However, with Guillain-Barré syndrome the immune system misidentifies the good as bad and targets the myelin sheath that surrounds the axons of many peripheral nerves, or even the axons themselves. These axons are the electrical wiring of the nerve cells which transport nerve signals and the destruction of their myelin sheath is much like scraping the insulation off your own home wiring, causing it to short. An axon's myelin sheath helps to ensure that a nervous system signal is able to travel the distance intact to the action location.

When certain diseases of the nerves' ravage myelin and the sheaths are vandalized, a victim's nerves become unable to transmit impulses correctly. When this happens, muscles and organs are not able to pick up accurate signals from the brain and carry out its orders. This communication works both ways as the brain is not only a command center but also a control center, receiving information such as touch, smell or various types of stress like heat, cold or exertion to modulate future commands sent out to the muscles and organs. With nervous system disorders the brain ends up receiving bad signal that manifests as numbness, tingling or painful sensations. The further a signal has to travel the more likely it is to be interrupted and degraded, making muscle weakness and tingling sensations to first be noticed in the distal hands and feet and then progress upwards in the arms and legs towards the neck and head.

From this description, one might conclude that all nervous system disorders are essentially alike. In a broad sense you could argue that point of view. Most nervous system disorders are nerve destructive disorders where a person's own immune system or genetic code turns on the victim. The differentiation comes from the trigger i.e. type of virus or genetic abnormality and the nomenclature of the disease. Amyotrophic lateral sclerosis (ALS), commonly known as Lou Gehrig's disease, is a neurodegenerative disease that is genetic. I'm sure if you ask a sufferer of either G-B or ALS if that matters they'd argue it makes no difference. Either person just wants it to stop so they can have their life back, though a G-B patient has much better odds of that than the 100% mortality rate of ALS.

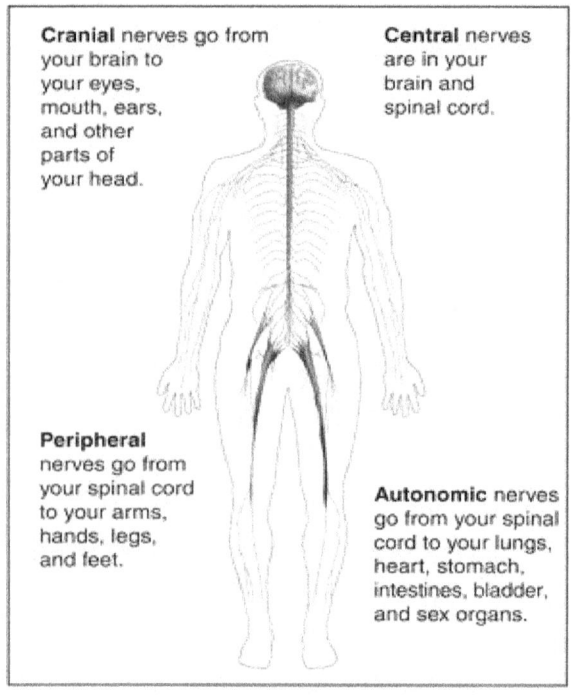

Cranial nerves go from your brain to your eyes, mouth, ears, and other parts of your head.

Central nerves are in your brain and spinal cord.

Peripheral nerves go from your spinal cord to your arms, hands, legs, and feet.

Autonomic nerves go from your spinal cord to your lungs, heart, stomach, intestines, bladder, and sex organs.

(PubMed Health No publication date expressed)[16]
The Four Divisions of the Human Nervous System

The victims of Guillain-Barre first notice a numbness or tingling of the hands and/or feet. They may have had a recent previous fever, bouts of fatigue, diarrhea or an upper respiratory tract infection a month or so prior to the numbness and tingling. From there, there is the rapid, progressive onset of muscle weakness as the peripheral nerves are affected. The weakness can be so debilitating as to essentially result in paralysis where the patient is unable to walk or lift their arms. At its worst in about 1 of 4 G-B victims, the disease weakens the respiratory muscles so much that the patient must be put on a ventilator to help them breathe and special attention paid to prevention of respiratory tract infections.

In about 60-70% of cases blood pressure and pulse rate are affected and become very erratic, bouncing between hypotension and hypertension, that is blood pressures so low that the patient may be near borderline shock or so high that there is a real risk of hemorrhage or an aneurysm, cerebral or otherwise.

Next on the hit parade of anything that can go wrong might go wrong list is loss of bowel control that may manifest as well, though thankfully such occurs in less than 10% of the cases. The cranial nerves that serve the swallow and chew mechanics may be involved thus the need for assistance with IV nutrition. Additionally, there may be gastrointestinal bleeds that must be treated, assuming that such a bleed is recognized in time which often only becomes suspected after lab work indicates an abnormally low blood cell count by way of hematocrit or hemoglobin testing. Bowel bleeds are then generally confirmed via a fecal occult test or endoscopy.

For those unlucky 1 in 5 or so who end up needing mechanical ventilation, the risk goes up substantially for pulmonary incidents such as pneumonia, upper respiratory tract infections and pulmonary (lung) emboli that can block off the arterial flow of basic life supporting oxygenated blood to the heart and brain. The fear of any bacterial infection that sets in the lungs is that it will progress from being localized to becoming systemic, resulting in septic shock. Supplemental oxygen may become necessary to overcome the loss of lung function, further complicating clinical efforts to maintain a safe blood Ph level. Too much O_2 can lead to the blood becoming alkaline ($\geq$7.45 Ph) and too little can result in the blood becoming acidic ($\leq$ 7.35), both not conducive to life unless addressed quickly with an adjustment in oxygen flow up or down. In extreme cases of low blood Ph where the threat to life is immediate, sodium bicarbonate, baking soda, is administered IV to help raise the Ph.

Reflexes are usually abnormal. It is not just the absence of a reflex response to a stimulus such as the hammer to the knee but also the presence of an exaggerated response to a stimuli as well. Some G-B patients are hypersensitive to touch to the point that a bed sheet on their skin causes excruciating pain.

Progression is usually rapid over a period of 2-5 days but can take as long as several weeks or as short as 8 hours and the debilitation may be as short as several days or as long as 6 months. The G-B syndrome by all accounts appears to be an equal opportunity disorder with no discernible preference for gender, race or age. In general, only about 1 out of 100,000 people experience this frightening syndrome. Most go on to fully recover but about 3-4% of patients decease during the recovery phase of the disease. About another quarter of those afflicted experience long term disability ranging from mild to severe, though very few are permanently incapacitated. Those most likely to face increased risk of death or long term severe disability are those who go into the disease process already compromised, which is often the elderly or those with other chronic conditions.

There can be multiple causes for a person to come down with Guillain-Barre. The most common cause is a previous infection by one of several bacterial or viral agents. The cytomegalovirus (CMV) is a part of the herpes family and is more common in underdeveloped nations and is found in regions with elevated population densities of low income and low education at rates approaching 100% of the population being seropositive for CMV antibodies. In more affluent and educated areas CMV antibodies are detectable in about 50 to 80% of the population with those over 80 years of age showing exposure rates near 90 %. CMV represents the most significant viral cause of birth defects in industrialized countries, in addition to being a culprit in G-B cases. (Wikipedia 2016) [17] There is good news regards a vaccine as a number of promising candidates are in mid to later stage testing though none is not yet ready for market.

Two other viruses associated with G-B syndrome are the varicella zoster (chicken pox) and Epstein-Barr virus, both variations of the herpes virus. There is a vaccine for the chicken pox virus but there is no vaccine for Epstein-Barr.

Epstein-Barr is implicated with mononucleosis, the Kissing Disease, and the outward singular observable sign is glandular swelling in the neck and other lymph node areas. This is the illness many of us know for how long it can last since many of its victims are laid up for 6-12 weeks due to severe fatigue. As with so many viruses, most of us would test positive for antibodies indicating we had been infected at one time or another but somehow managed to stay sign and symptom free. Ignorance, indeed, can be bliss.

Chicken pox has also been connected to triggering cases of G-B and the worst that most of us infected with this virus experienced was the aesthetically displeasing pustules. Unfortunately, having chicken pox leaves us vulnerable to shingles (herpes zoster) later in life when the chicken pox virus manifests itself along our nerve pathways as inflamed pustules and is incredibly painful. To add insult to injury, the accompanying scabbing and eruptions are enough to force people to avoid social situations due to their appearance. There is a vaccine for both chicken pox and shingles.

Another nasty that can trigger G-B syndrome is Campylobacter jejuni. *C. jejuni* is a bacteria found in the livestock industry ranging from poultry to cattle. It is also found in wild bird populations and waterways and is one of the reasons our governments insist on pasteurization of milk. For those who have it in their tiny skulls that unpasteurized milk is perfectly safe for their children and somehow magically infers super powers upon them, that is true only in so far as *C. jejuni* is rarely fatal. However, a *C. jejuni* infection can leave a person with a very nasty case of gastroenteritis manifested as severe abdominal cramps and explosive diarrhea. Considering the position of a freshened cow's udder to the bathroom along with my own experience on dairy farms in Wisconsin, I have zero faith that purveyors of unpasteurized milk can maintain an uncontaminated milk supply by hand and cow teat washing alone.

Mycoplasma pneumoniae is a bacteria that also may trigger an episode of G-B. For many years, it was thought that *M. pneumoniae* was not a bacteria but a virus. With the advent of widespread penicillin antibiotic production and use during WWII, *M. pneumoniae* was being considered more strongly as a virus since it did not respond to treatment with penicillin and war research efforts seemed to support this idea. It wasn't until 1963 that scientists nailed down the bug to being a bacteria and not a virus. If you've ever heard the term 'walking pneumoniae' it would be in reference to this lung infection. (Wikipedia 2015)[18]

Vaccines have been accused of triggering cases of G-B but that is a red herring and no relationship has ever been established, yet rumors and misinformation persist much to the chagrin of family doctors.

The only treatments for G-B is immunoglobulin therapy or plasma exchange through a process called plasmapharesis. Plasmapharesis is a process where red and white blood cells are separated from one another and then the plasma portion, the milky yellow liquid portion of the blood, is discarded and the red blood cells returned. The idea behind plasmapharesis is the destructive antibodies attacking the nervous system in their misguided quest are lessened in number thus reducing their overall destructive power.

With immunoglobulin therapy patients receive ultra high doses of various proteins that normally assist the immune system in carrying out its duties. How or why exactly this rallies and organizes a more appropriate immune response is not fully understood. As with so much of medicine, we know certain treatments or compounds work but are not certain of the specific cause and effect, though in defense we often know enough to grasp the big picture and argue cogently for this or that use or method.

Another line of treatment for G-B involves the use of corticosteroids, a class of drugs that have all sorts of wonderful properties to combat immune disorders and inflammations. They are used to treat conditions as wide ranging as skin rashes, such as poison ivy, by calming down the body's immune response that creates the swelling, itch and burn of the skin, and brain tumors to help suppress cerebral swelling and edema. Other conditions treated with corticosteroids are lung disorders such as chronic obstructive pulmonary disorder (COPD), ulcerative colitis, Crohn's disease, lupus and arthritis. In fact, there probably isn't an autoimmune disease where prednisone or dexamethasone cannot theoretically play some sort of role, though prescribing of corticosteroids is done with caution since there are some worrisome side effects.

Vaccines are often accused of being a trigger for Guillain-Barre. Then again, vaccines are accused of everything from causing autism to forgetting your wife's anniversary. We know Guillain-Barre "….is a rare, acute autoimmune disease of the peripheral nervous system that is characterized by rapidly advancing, bilateral, ascending motor neuron paralysis that usually occurs after an acute respiratory or gastrointestinal infection. On rare occasions, GBS manifests after vaccination. It is the leading cause of acute paralysis in developed countries and remains the most reported serious adverse event after trivalent influenza vaccination in the Vaccine Adverse Event Reporting System (VAERS) data base. This data base has a report rate of 0.70 per 1 million vaccinations. The incidence rate of GBS in the general population is 0.6 to 4.0 cases per 100,000 persons per year; the typical rate of GBS in recipients of any vaccine is 0.07 to 0.46 cases per 100,000 persons." (Wang, et al.)[19]

Of course vaccines can have side effects. The triad of side effects taught to every nursing, pharmacy and medical student for exams that challenge students to name the side effects of X medication is headache, fever or nausea. The most common side effect for vaccines delivered by injection is redness, itching or soreness at the injection site and that's likely as much to do with the quality of the needle as it is with the compound itself. There is nothing like the drama of vaccination day when a school gym is filled with 6 year olds who are convinced they are about to be fatally impaled.

The incidence of serious life threatening side effects from vaccines according to the previously mentioned VAERES database referenced on the preceding page is pegged at between 0.7-4.6 per million regards influenza vaccines. Adverse events for all vaccines have reports of 10,000-20,000 per 10 million shots administered, meaning a range of 1 event per 500 to 1 per 1000 shots. The VAERES database makes it explicitly clear that the reports it receives should not be considered reliable in and of itself as many health professionals have varying personal criteria for what they think is an adverse event worth reporting. Some report nearly every sniffle while others may not consider it worth the effort to submit a report unless a patient is hospitalized, making VAERS a passive reporting system.(VAERES-Vaccine Adverse Events)[20]

Now that we understand G-B can be triggered by an autoimmune response where confused antibodies are likely set in motion by the in vivo presence of the Zika virus or some sort of other pathogen, it adds to the overall concern and confusion that the current outbreak is indeed something to sweat. While it is not known if the virus itself invades the neurons or simply somehow tricks immune system antibodies into misidentifying neurons for targeted destruction, it doesn't much matter at this point.

What is making everyone from WHO/PAHO so nervous is that as of February 2016 Brazil, Columbia, Venezuela and El Salvador are showing frighteningly high spikes in G-B. A direct cause cannot be stated and part of the problem is that Zika is only detectable for about 2-7 days within the body, meaning that once someone does show up exhibiting G-B signs and symptoms, a month or more has usually passed. That both the Zika epidemic and spikes in G-B are showing up together is just too likely to be more than coincidence and it would be malpractice to make the claim that there is no connection or to excuse inaction of definitively determining a link, or not, between the two. Any indifference to a Guillain-Barre to Zika connection would be a sort of paralysis in of itself that must be avoided. For now, it is only responsible to take seriously the correlation between the Latin America Zika outbreak and dramatic spike in Guillain-Barre cases.

Microcephaly

Microcephaly simply is medical jargon for small head. There are competing definitions of what comprises a diagnosis of microcephaly. One definition is that the head must be outside of two standard deviations while another prefers to define it as outside of three standard deviations. Still another prefers to define microcephaly as a head circumference that is $\leq$ 31.48 cm for a newborn and in the lower 3 percentile or those in the $\leq$5 percentile range with a circumference $\leq$ 32.14. Some are more stringent still using a 1 percentile cutoff. A median sized head on a newborn is 35.8 cm per CDC growth charts. (CDC, 2001)[21]

The head makes the person. Take the head away and what is left is called an anonymous corpse. Take an arm or leg away and you still have a person. Even a dead person with a head is more 'alive' than a body without a head. During the Tudor reigns that included Henry VIII, it was acutely and widely understood that notification a person was about to lose their head meant the poor soul was going to lose their entire identity and essence once their head was separated from their body. Suicides would sometimes have their heads separated from their bodies by church authorities to supposedly prevent the suicide from being able to enter the Kingdom of God, just in case to make sure there were no mix ups about who was allowed in or out. For good measure, civil and church authorities may have further mutilated the suicide corpse. Also, during the Middle Ages, suicide was often equated with murder or even diabolical possession in various parts of Europe, so two other penalties besides beheading of the corpse also were sometimes enforced, namely confiscation of property and refusal of burial in consecrated grounds.

Decapitation, or beheading, was performed not as a means of providing for a more humane death but as a legal expression that the convicted's crime was as most vulgar and reprehensible imaginable. An order to take someone's head was about as high of an expression of authoritarian disdain that could be administered. It also sent a message about who was really in charge. After a slave revolt in the US in 1811, about one hundred slaves had their heads removed, many of them stuck on pikes within sight of other slaves to warn them to not get any ideas. I'm sure there was no miscommunication of intent judging by the relatively docile demeanor of the slave population prior to the Civil War.

I think I've established that having a head attached to a body is certainly more aesthetically pleasing and civilized plus a basic requirement for life. Your head has a face by which everyone recognizes you and you recognize everyone else. We are quite keen on miniscule differences between heads, quick to note any asymmetry such as one ear being larger than the other or a nose too small or too large in proportion to the rest of the face. Eyes that are set wide or narrow may indicate disease in the womb and a forehead too high or absent casts suspicion on intelligence. Of course, it is perfectly possible to have an asymmetrical feature and be perfectly normal and most such people are wonderfully normal. For good or ill, a lack of symmetry in a person's head raises concern over that person's competence, trustworthiness or state of health.

Anomalies of human anatomy have a tragic history by today's social mores and standards where most nations now go to great lengths to bring the disabled into the fold of the mainstream society. A couple of centuries ago having a club foot, being blind, deaf or mute, limbless, or two of something where one of something should be was a good way to be cast out to the edges of society if not outright killed. Many such tragic souls were purloined into forced labor, or their own personal circumstances made so desperate they were vulnerable to depraved manipulations.

All sorts of human malformations were paraded in front of the public, macabre spectacles people would pay to see, to insult and even to physically abuse. There was Jojo the Dogfaced Boy who suffered from excessive body hair (hirusutism) and Lobster Boy with his deformed hands and feet. Caterpillar Man, who was limbless, was a well known attraction amongst many others. One of the more famous freaks was a fellow named Mordake who endured the condition of living with what is referred to as a parasitic twin. In this case, his parasitic twin was an extra face plastered upon his head said to mimic Mordake's own facial expressions. He succumbed to suicide after a short life of being a social outcast.

Included in this troupe of freak theater were those who suffered from microcephalic birth defects. If you are familiar with the character of Zippy the Pinhead by Bill Griffith, a comic strip that was syndicated in 1976, Zippy is allegedly based on a resemblance to a person afflicted with microcephaly. However, changing sensibilities within the American public eventually led to Zippy returning to the underground culture from whence it came, much to the chagrin of fans and much to the relief of those who thought it minimized and mocked those with disabilities.

Microcephaly is now being thrust back into national and

international consciousness by the outburst of Zika virus in Central and South Americas. It has been observed that cases of reported microcephaly in infants have spiked considerably in Zika affected areas, especially Brazil with similar reports showing a similar corresponding rise of microcephaly in Columbia and Venezuela.

Once again, though, just as with Guillain-Barre, WHO and PAHO emphasize that they cannot present us with a definitive cause and effect between the virus and the particular birth defect of microcephaly. And, again, further complicating matters is the short time window in which a positive test for Zika can be conducted, 2-7 days.

The precise mechanisms that produce a small brained fetus or infant are often opaque, though piece by piece the window is clearing. Microcephaly has many known causes that must be considered as legitimate candidates ranging from teratogenics, environmental substances that cause birth defects, like lead or methyl mercury a mother is exposed to while pregnant, or chromosomal and genetic abnormalities such as Trisomy 18 or 21 where there is a third copy of the material from the chromosome. Additionally, certain viral diseases such as rubella (mumps) can be a microcephaly trigger.

The typical cranial vault of the adult ranges between 60 to 90 cubic inches with males being only slightly larger than females. Brain weight comes in at almost 3 pounds exactly. Large headed people do have larger brains and the speculation is that the extra capacity is needed for autonomic and somatic functions, no different than a heavier vehicle may need more horsepower to run at its best. IQ wise there is no known benefit or drawback to having a slightly larger or smaller brain than average, though in the 19th century a few scientists offered up that there was a direct correlation between head size and intelligence, a hypothesis that has been debunked.

Brain weight ratios of other species through the animal

kingdom, the ratio of brain weight to body weight is: for fish, 1:5000; for reptiles it is about 1:1500; for birds, 1:220; for most mammals, 1:180, and for humans, 1:50. (Purves, Dale)[22] These ratios hold up to be fairly accurate across all species in determining general intellectual capacity.

We obsess over the brain and its capacity. The most accepted ways for measuring intelligence are through various means of testing we believe to be objective. However, any person serious about such a subject knows that in examining the contents and methods of the various tests used to judge quality of intelligence, or quantify it, knows that there are serious and severe cultural and personal biases built in by the limits of the test creators own life experience and learning. A person who grows up in New York City has a far different life experience than a person who grows up along the Louisiana Gulf Coast. Intimate, detailed knowledge of ocean and shoreline habitats, boats and weather are valuable to a Gulf of Mexico fisherman or other ocean-side based resident. Someone from New York City finds such knowledge, at best, to be trivial. Even in tests that involve what on the surface looks like pure mathematics can be biased, with a person with a prejudice against decimals and percentages used in banking and finance maybe believing that fractions and formulas are better due to their own familiarity with carpentry or the other skilled trades. Tests offer insight into the test givers and creators more deeply than those who take them.

My favorite test was one given to students in Catholic Catechism Direction classes (CCD) we were required to attend on Wednesday nights during the school year. In that test, we were given the scenario of nuclear Armageddon but had the good fortune of a heads up it was coming so we could plan for how we would use our resources and who we'd allow in to our limited space radioactive proof bomb shelter. There are several scenarios to this game in which what is described about each person is a skill or occupation along with a character judgment of prostitute, dropout, priest, policeman, etc. Of course, we were expected to make room for the priest and nun and toss out Dixie the stripper and the bossy pants cop. That is an extreme example of how tests reflect the values of the test giver more than the test taker since the test creators confined our choices to one's of their choosing. In not so dissimilar ways, Zika pregnancies are about to test our value systems on an individual and social basis.

Earlier I mentioned that head size has no known correlation to intelligence and that is true but only true when the cranium in question falls within normal, healthy ranges. A cranial vault half the size of what is age appropriate is guaranteed to have a compromised mind. A microcephalic infant has a brain-body weight ratio between 1:100 and 1:150, one third to one half the size it should be which is 1:50 brain to body weight.

The biggest clue to how Zika may hold back brain development is the cytomegalovirus, which is known to be a cause of disability in about 1 out 750 births and for which there is no cure or vaccine. We know that CMV attacks developing neurons during the first trimester, possibly destroying the stem cells that give rise to cerebral neurons. The brain's scaffolding is also attacked, meaning that there is no structure or only a deformed foundation for neurons to build on, further messing things up.

Since testing is only possible within the window of 2-7 days while enough of a Zika viral load is present and 75% of Zika infected persons display no symptoms, it is highly unlikely that evidence of such an infection will be caught to give a heads up about a possible birth defect. Testing for Zika antibodies is highly problematic as well since Zika comes across as looking like dengue or chikungunya, reducing the diagnosis to a process of elimination that is time consuming, inexact and expensive.

The first test for the making of a diagnosis of

microcephaly can be made during pregnancy by means of ultrasound to view developmental progress, but this is not possible until around the second trimester, 18 to 20 weeks in and almost half way through the gestation period of 40 weeks.

Enough of the brain does manage to develop to give rise to a human that is able to survive and perform basic functions. Like any disability, there is a range of severity that can be quantified or qualified. Most children with microcephaly are special needs children for life who will need various amounts of medical attention. In addition to cognitive deficits that are insurmountable there will be physiological issues that will be insurmountable ranging from fine motor control, vision and hearing issues to possibly being wheel chair bound and oblivious of surroundings. Some microcephalic children are able to integrate with a limited amount of success but most are bound to their families or institutions for life with no hope of achieving an appreciable amount of independence. Maybe worst of all, they cannot expect to have a normal lifespan, only one that is about 20 to 40% of the normal life span of 80 years for US citizens. Just when you think such news couldn't get any worse, it does.

The same Zika virus that looks to be the blame for microcephaly may also be able to cause anencephaly, a more severe and damaging neuronal birth defect. Anencephaly is a failure of the neural tube to close properly during a fetus's development. The narrow channel within the neural tube is supposed to flap over and close during the first 21 to 28 days of pregnancy to establish the embryo's spinal cord and brain. What also happens when the cranial end of the neural tube fails to close is an absence of a major portion of the brain, skull, and scalp. Those born with this malformation come into this world without the front part of their brain and a cerebrum, the thinking and coordinating part of the brain. The rest of the brain tissue is sometimes exposed, minus the skull cover or skin. An infant born with anencephaly is likely to be deaf, blind, unconscious and unable to feel or respond to pain. Some infants birthed with anencephaly may possess only a primitive and incomplete brain stem. Finally, the lack of a properly functioning cerebrum forever eliminates self awareness.

An infant with microcephaly may exhibit a high-pitched cry, poor feeding, convulsions, increased movement of the arms and legs (spasticity), hyperactivity, developmental delays and mental retardation. As the child grows older, his or her face continues to grow while the skull does not. This causes the child to develop a disproportionately large face, a receding forehead and a loose, often wrinkled scalp. The rest of the body is often underweight and proportionately smaller than normal.

Breathing and other reflexive responses to touch, sound, heat or cold may or may not be able to be elicited with probing. Such an infant is often not even a suitable organ donor as other organs are often impacted as well. ("Anencephaly Information Page: National Institute of Neurological Disorders and Stroke (NINDS)", 2015)[23]

One researcher, Marli Tenório, an infectious disease expert at the Aggeu Magalhães Research Center of Brazil's Pernambuco state, tested the spinal fluid of a dozen microcephalic infants and found definitive evidence Zika was present in all 12. Again, PAHO is issuing a serious caution to not cite these findings as proven link. Of many of the reported cases of microcephaly in Brazil, the heightened attention has created a circumstance of an increase in reports that may have not occurred before news of the outbreak. To the Brazil Health Ministry's credit, they have dutifully investigated these reports to winnow out those case where other causes are at work. Of the several thousand suspected cases at this point, many have been dismissed as not being microcephaly. What they've been left with as likely or highly likely cases is still alarming in that what used to be 10 cases a year of microcephaly is now 10 per week as of early February, 2016.

New methods of testing for Zika include testing for Immunoglobin M in cerebral spinal fluid which shows up as a response to Zika antibodies. Img M hangs around in CSF for several weeks, creating a larger window to make a diagnosis of exposure to the virus. It also is evidence that Zika is making its way into the nervous system. ("PBS", 2016)[24]

Microcephaly is not a trivial birth defect hence the heavy handwringing that is going on by American governments and how to deal with this as a health crisis. The rise in cases and connection with Zika are not mere speculation anymore. There is ample enough evidence that a strategy needs to be put together to deal with this problem and there is ample evidence we really don't have one.

Ticking Time Bomb

The virus is on the march. The United States has suitable habitat for *A. aegypti* and *A. albopictus* extending as far west as 200 miles west of the Mississippi River and as far north as the Ohio Valley, plus scattered areas in California, Oregon, Wisconsin and Minnesota. Already the virus has been documented leaving Brazil and traveling north into Colombia, Venezuela, El Salvador, Nicaragua and Mexico plus the Caribbean. As the weather warms into the spring and summer seasons, mosquitoes will become more active in the United States and travelers from the southern countries will arrive back in the US, unwittingly infected and themselves a vector of Zika into the US mosquito population which in turn will infect US citizens. And so the cycle will go.

No one knows how many people are going to be infected. Anything is a guesstimate as of this moment. What we can tell is that the virus is moving rapidly through the southern global populations, giving us a clue as to how fast it will spread in the habitat range of the two types of mosquito that spread the virus.

My own estimate is 4 million in the US could be infected

by the winter of 2016-17 in the United States. The state likely to be most hard hit is Florida, about the worst possible place for such an outbreak to happen thanks in no small part to Florida's refusal to expand and extend health insurance to its residents. It is a well known fact that people, even when sick or at high risk for one thing or another, avoid seeing the doctor precisely to avoid going into debt they may not be able to handle. This is a recipe for a disaster especially as it is regards expectant mothers and other parents who may be considering starting a family.

We know that only 1 of 4 people infected display signs or symptoms of Zika infection, meaning that 3 of 4 will have no clue they are infected and they will be at higher risk of transmitting the disease by having themselves get mosquito bit, unprotected sex or even by donating blood or plasma. As of now, there is no simple mass testing that can be done on the blood and plasma supplies.

However, per the Plasma Protein Therapeutics Association, flaviviruses like the West Nile (NV), dengue, yellow fever and Japanese encephalitis viruses have a similar lipid envelope to that of the Zika virus. The relatively large size of the virus and its lipid envelope makes it highly susceptible to steps with virus inactivation and removal capacity used during the manufacturing processes, such as solvent-detergent (S/D), low pH incubation, caprylate, pasteurization or dry-heat treatments, nanofiltration or fractionation processes. The effectiveness of these processes has been demonstrated on other lipid-enveloped model viruses which are quite similar to Zika virus, namely the bovine viral diarrhea virus (BVDV) or tick-borne encephalitis virus (TBEV), and most importantly the West Nile virus, another flavivirus which is even more closely related to the Zika virus. (PPTA, "Plasma Protein Therapeutics Association", 2016)[25]

Blood and plasma donors would be near impossible to screen since every person is exposed nearly daily to mosquito activity of one sort or another.   It would be impossible to stop blood and plasma donations and attempt to import blood products from non threatened areas of the globe due to logistics and shelf life of blood product.

Manufacturers of blood products are very confident their processes to protect the blood and plasma supplies are more than sufficient to avoid putting contaminated product out on the market. This is based entirely not on actually testing the process against Zika infected samples, but by comparison with viruses similar in size and structure. What they are saying, per Plasma Protein Therapeutics Association is, 'Our safety processes work on that and that so it will work on this'.

That's a fine argument to make as a prognostication but it is still exactly that—a prediction. It is not an actual test that is observed, recorded, challenged by other researchers and peer reviewed by outside disinterested third parties. Then again, it certainly isn't reasonable to shut down an entire blood and plasma supply industry that is critical to patient care. At the end of the day, there is no choice but to hope, confidently I believe, that the current processes for blood products are adequate safe guards.

Yet, we've had warnings in the past and paid dearly for not heeding them with haste.   There was the HIV contamination of the blood supply that adversely impacted many patients who were not high risk until they had the misfortune of needing a couple of pints. Hepatitis C, a liver destroying virus, was also passed through the blood supply and only indirectly tested for by measuring a liver enzyme called ALT (alanine aminotransferase) that becomes elevated when high Hep C viral loads are present. It was not until the 1990's that a direct test for Hep C was developed and able to be applied on a mass scale to donated blood. Sadly, our current Hepatitis C crisis in the United States, approximately 5 million infected, is due in no small part to tainted blood products that slipped through the indirect ALT testing method.

The most high risk patients for a contaminated blood product with Zika would be a pregnant women early in her gestational period of the first trimester or someone who is immunocompromised in some way. Obviously, anyone receiving a blood product is already in a bit of pickle health wise so you can see how this starts to become a problem. Patients that would normally survive and go on to thrive thanks to a blood product, might instead find they have been kicked hard enough while down to not be able to fully recuperate. And without testing in the 2-7 day window we currently have for Zika, doctors and patients may have no idea that Zika is even part of a problem since fever, joint pain and malaise are symptoms so common as to be present in hundreds of maladies.

Initially, many US health experts dismissed Zika as a minor threat at most, claiming only those people who have travelled outside of the country to Brazil had anything at all to be concerned about, and even then any infectious result of a mosquito encounter was likely to go unnoticed and without complication. Now many of those same health personnel are pedaling backwards a bit, stating that we can't say with any certainty the United States will not have a problem on its hands in the summer of 2016, that there are just too many variables.

As of the first week of February 2016, health officials are discovering that Zika is present in not only blood, but saliva and urine as well, contradicting previous reports that there was no chance of Zika being present in either saliva or urine. The report out of Dallas of Zika being passed via sex prompted a reconsideration of how the virus can be transmitted. It is inevitable we may have to revise the risk profile regards saliva and urine being possible reservoirs by which a casual encounter with either fluid may pose a risk.

The initial reports of live virus being discovered in urine and saliva came from Brazil's Oswaldo Cruz Foundation in anticipation of the annual 5 day Carnival celebration preceding the Ash Wednesday kick off of the Lenten season. Since Carnival can be summed as being a bacchanal event where partiers bathe themselves in copious amounts of alcohol, normal inhibitions are reduced and saliva and urine flow quite freely on and into places normally not associated with either expectorant. Brazilian health officials correctly anticipated the celebration as a good reason to test urine and saliva to see if they should give everyone a head's up. Disappointingly, they did indeed find live virus. ("Los Angeles Times", 2016)[26]

As US travelers to South America return home, there is no feasible or plausible way to determine if their presence in the general public square poses a risk. Specifically, they do not since what we know is that Zika is not spread by easy casual contact or is airborne like say the influenza virus. Also, it is entirely realistic to classify such travelers as low risk human to human transmitters in light of the known, that being even if a person is infected they are unlikely to have any health problems. However, such travelers from infected geographic areas are not without posing problems.

As more unwittingly infected travelers from South America enter the United States, the higher the risk of widespread contagion as the Zika mosquitoes *A. aegypti* and *A. albopictus* sink their drill-like proboscises into the skin of South American visitors to the US for that all important protein rich blood meal needed for egg production. At first blush, one might think there aren't that many South American travelers to the US but that would be inaccurate.

Between 2004 and 2011 Brazil alone was a port of egress of annual U.S. arrivals that increased by 292 percent, from 385,000 to 1,508,000. Recent economic problems in Brazil has reduced the number of Brazilian tourists from the 2011 number by about a third, the latest peak year with a hard statistic documenting such travel. Each traveler on average stayed for a period of time of about 16 days, plenty of time to get out and about and travel many miles from their port of entry. As you might guess, Miami is the single largest port of entry for arrivals from all over South America. (Riker, "Journal of International Commerce and Economics", 2013)[27]

One million people annually is not a trivial number. That's a rough estimate and it is only a rough estimate for those from Brazil. Throw in the other South and Central American countries and that number goes up to as high as 20 million annual visitors, including Mexico. As it stands now, the high infection rate areas are Brazil, Columbia and Venezuela but there notable reports of Zika infection in Mexico, El Salvador and Nicaragua per PAHO and the trend is on a steady, fast upward climb in those countries that is unlikely to slow unless a Black Swan type of event occurs that is detrimental to the mosquito population, or human intervention manages to knock down the mosquito population.

The highest months of travel for international travelers according to the US Dept of Commerce are usually December and January over the Christmas holiday. The next highest month is July, prime time for mosquito populations to be active and in high breeding season throughout the entire United States. Spring and summer months are also the heavy traffic times for migrant workers, especially farm workers who enter the US to work the fields and follow planting and harvest seasons as they move north along with the warming weather.

As you can see, there is no shortage of available targets for our two Zika mosquitoes to lite upon as they search for the next harvest. The question that remains to be answered is how fast will there be a spread of the virus through the immunologically naïve US population. No one as of yet has put forth a number where they think a critical mass will be reached that makes Zika a permanent part of the disease landscape that must be addressed annually. Judging by the numbers of travelers and numbers of known infections in Brazil alone, I'd wager that 2016 is the year Zika becomes a permanent part of the US infectious disease landscape. Zika's easy route of transmission coupled with the fact that most infected persons have no clue they are even a carrier capable of spreading Zika further amongst mosquitoes, or possibly by intimate human contact amongst each other, is the perfect covert method for Zika to insinuate itself into the larger population.

Some infectious disease experts consider the likelihood of a widespread Zika problem remote based on how other flaviviruses such as West Nile, yellow fever and dengue have behaved within the United States. According to the CDC, in 2015 there were 2060 cases of West Nile. Dengue virus has had very limited incursions into the United States with outbreaks limited to small geographical areas such as Hawaii in 2001, Brownsville Texas in 2005 and Monroe County (Key West) Florida in 2009-2011. All three outbreaks were self limiting, meaning they dissipated on their own without some sort of massive intervention. Hawaii's cases numbered about 120 while Brownsville had only about 25. The Monroe County, FL outbreak was notable for the length of time of two years while the other two outbreaks were only a few months long. During that time, the Keys yielded only about 90 cases. (Adalja et al, " Emerging Infectious Disease journal - CDC", 2012)[28]

Based on how the flavivirus outbreaks of dengue and West Nile have behaved, infectious disease specialists are not exactly running through the streets lighting their hair on fire to get us to pay attention to an impending apocalypse. By no stretch of the imagination do they consider such outbreaks irrelevant and they are keeping close tabs as well as they can. Puerto Rico now has annual dengue events and in numbers large enough that they can issue charts displaying current or recent outbreaks with historical averages. Puerto Rico keeps it annual case numbers around several hundred but there have been years where up to 25,000 dengue infections have been reported per the CDC.

The conditions for dengue, yellow fever and chikungunya are not generally favorable north of the southern US border. West Nile, however, has managed to do just fine in all 48 continental United States, each summer bringing a peak in cases about August. Based on this history, health officials are cautiously optimistic that Zika will be limited as well. Then again, based on how the West Nile virus has spread like a wave from the East Coast to the West Coast over the US since 2004, the same health officials are crossing their fingers, praying that the worst case scenario does not play out.

Louisiana continues to have mandatory reporting for any suspected cases of yellow fever, its historic memory advising the state that they are vulnerable should they forget the major epidemics that swept through New Orleans and killed over a 1,000 citizens in 1905. After that, serious mosquito eradication efforts occurred along with development of a vaccine in the 1930's. Chances are you know very few people, if any, who have been vaccinated against yellow fever, the 19th century scourge that killed tens of thousands in the United States as far north as New York. Today, the only US citizens who have been vaccinated for yellow fever tend to be travelers to equatorial South America and Africa, a requirement of entry is to show proof of vaccination by presenting a Yellow Card.

Considering the size of the United States and the fact there is no vaccine for Zika and likely will be no vaccine until at least 2017, and even that is optimistic, mosquito eradication efforts will likely be spotty. Naturally, considering the receptive state of certain sectors of the US population to hyperbolic assumption, fueled in large part by muckraking news outlets, there will be demands that everything possible be done with widespread misinformation that any chemical interventions for eradication will be too risky. Not to leave out reactionaries opposed to most government programs, there will be financial and budgetary claims blown out of proportion to justify a 'wait and see' plan, one that will only be implemented when one too many citizens is found to be seriously infected. The question really is: What is our tolerance level for total numbers of seriously ill patients found to be victimized by Zika.

Certain areas are more prone to infectious outbreaks, namely urban areas due to the close proximity of people and mosquito. More rural areas may be more swampy and have more standing water but the lack of density of human populations breaks the chain of mosquito biting an actively infected person and transmitting further. It is a simple math of opportunity.

The single largest problem is the Zika virus taking hold and determining what to do with women of childbearing age. Already the CDC and NIH are cautioning potential mothers to take steps to reduce their possible exposure when traveling and advising that women trying to get pregnant or are pregnant should exercise caution in areas where Zika outbreaks are present in high density, namely the Central and South American countries plus the Caribbean islands.

The ticking time bomb we have is, geographically speaking, sitting straight south the United States. As 2016 progresses we are at risk of a slow rolling explosion and disaster that will rock our health system from south to north. Optimism is a wonderful thing but too often it can be detrimental in the sense that it allows ourselves to downplay risk and make the bad bet, ignoring taking steps toward proper precautions to have a solid Plan B in place, let alone a solid Plan A.

Pregnancy & Birth Defects

If Zika is a ticking time bomb, pregnancy is ground zero where the most damage will be done. Every year within the United States about 6.5 million pregnancies occur. Out of that number about 4.25 million result in a live birth. A little math shows us that approximately 2.25 million pregnancies end annually due to miscarriage, abortion or spontaneous premature birth. About 40% of all pregnancies within the United States are unintended. Total pregnancies would be a city two and a half times the size of the city of Chicago (about 2.8 million per the US Census Bureau Quick Facts). With numbers that size, pregnancy is a major life event that is an economy all its own.

The single largest concern ahead of all other worries regards Zika is how the virus affects pregnancy. Teratology is the study of birth defects and their causes and Zika certainly has captured the interest of teratologists. While we know that there are a number of causes which contribute to birth defects and infant mortality, many still aren't 100% convinced there is a definitive cause and effect between Zika and birth defects. The circumstantial evidence is overwhelming and the correlation too strong to ignore. Still, making all of this concern more problematic is the difficulty in testing to pin down a Zika smoking gun due to the 2-7 day window. In the end, what we end up with is a system where risk or cause is concluded by ruling out other things like diseases or toxins such as syphilis, toxoplasmosis, rubella, cytomegalovirus or herpes simplex virus. None of the other flaviviruses are known causes of birth defects, still again leaving room for serious doubts and questions.

The best cause and effect Zika link there is now is a health history from the mother. If a fetus or infant is determined to have microcephaly, the doctor looking for a connection would ask the mother if she had signs or symptoms of a Zika infection such as rash, fatigue, conjunctivitis or joint pain and when. As of this writing, these observations are being made in Brazil and the emerging pattern is in about 75% of cases mothers who gave birth to microcephalic infants are reporting recollections of such Zika signs and symptoms during their pregnancies. The gestation dates are ranging from 6 weeks up to 20 weeks during the pregnancy, though the grain of salt in such a number is the imperfection of human memory.

The CDC has done tissue analysis from two infants with microcephaly who both died one day after being born. Other testing of tissue came from two miscarriages. Each of the samples came from the state of Rio Grande do Norte in Brazil where the Zika outbreak is at the worst. Each of the mothers reported in their health histories of having a rash associated with a Zika virus infection and that the rash appeared during the first trimester of pregnancy. However, none of the mothers were tested for Zika infection during the golden 2-7 day window.

Each of the four specimens collected tested positive for the Zika virus RNA by testing that used PCR, polymerase chain reaction. PCR testing is done with snips from two different areas of the viral RNA strands. Viral antigens in two of the four samples were found by using stained viral antibodies which pointed to evidence of Zika in one of the placental tissue samples and one of the brain sample tissues.   Four samples of tissue with no direct observed evidence but Zika positive is not proof positive but it does provide a foundation.(Schuler-Faccini, 2016)[29]

In his virology blog, Vincent Racaniello, a Higgins Professor in the Department of Microbiology and Immunology at Columbia University's College of Physicians and Surgeons, writes that he thinks the clinching study, "Zika Virus Associated with Microcephaly" was made in the New England Journal Medicine in an article published February 10, 2016 by Jernej Mlakar, M.D and colleagues.

Racaniello summarizes the NEJM study, and two other studies findings, writing:

"Here is the clincher – the entire Zika virus genome was identified in brain tissue by next-generation sequencing! Analysis of the sequence revealed 99.7% nucleotide identity with a Zika virus strain isolated from a patient from French Polynesia in 2013, and a strain from Sao Paulo from 2015. These findings agree with the hypothesis that the current Brazilian outbreak was triggered by a virus from Asia.

Up to now there have been few data that strongly link Zika virus infection to congenital birth defects. Of these three new studies, the recovery of a full length Zika virus genome from an infant with microcephaly is the most convincing. Given the rapidity by which new data are emerging, it seems likely that additional evidence demonstrating that Zika virus can cause microcephaly will soon be forthcoming." (Racaniello, 2016)[30]

Racaniello lays out his case and has the chops to make it stick. The data gathered previously was not able to stand on its own nor was it at a point, when put together, to be considered damning. Racaniello is laying claim that there is now enough evidence that if any worry was being tempered by cautious optimism, that there was no connection between Zika and birth defect, that doubt should be gone.

Zika appears to do damage pretty much the same way as the cytomegalovirus does in that the neural tube is targeted and then damaged in such a way that prevents the neural tube from folding back on itself to close up. With the neural tube failure to close, the rest of the fetal brain fails to develop. The developing fetal skull responds to the lack of brain mass by growing only enough to cover the seriously underdeveloped brain, thus the missing top of the head.

It is at around week 5 at the beginning of the embryonic period where tissue that will grow into a nervous system is present. This is during the period referred to as differentiation where cells will start developing into other major bodily systems. If there is a cell specific toxin present, some other foreign assault or a deficiency, these tissues can be vulnerable to all sorts of damage. One that many mothers are aware of is that a lack of folic acid, part of the B vitamin group, may put their child at risk for Spinal Bifida, a debilitating birth defect where the neural tube fails to close and the baby is born without a normal spinal cord. The brain may or may not be affected.

Birth defects are less common today than in previous decades. Very much like how certain diseases are distant memories thanks to vaccination programs, birth defects are uncommon enough that many of us probably have a hard time naming an affected person or family. But the threat is still there in about 3% of all births. The only reason there is less of a threat is dedicated prenatal programs and education efforts along with strict regulation of various teratogenic substances, especially household and workplace chemicals ranging from household cleaners to agricultural pesticides and herbicides.

Vaccination programs have dramatically altered the birth

defect total. The 1969 introduction of the Rubella vaccine was the last great step in reducing birth defects, meaning that a one step intervention on a mass scale provided such dramatic benefits. Other childhood vaccination programs have made pregnancy later in life less risky for both mother and fetus. Unfortunately, there is no vaccine or treatment for a Zika infected mother and, if one should appear soon, it may well be something that can only be done well prior to pregnancy, not during. The medical establishment is quite skittish about drugs and vaccines being given to pregnant women until they are absolutely convinced that the benefit outweighs the potential for harm by an almost ridiculously unrealistic ratio.

The most common birth defect is the class of congenital heart defects that may affect heart valves or other structure of the heart. About one in 110 infants is diagnosed with a congenital heart issue. Fortunately, strides in neonate and in vivo surgery have yielded satisfying results in resolving many of these defects. Still, about 20% of infants with a major birth defect succumb.

Following is a list of 21 major defects from the Centers for Disease Control and Prevention--Birth Defects, the instances of occurrence and totals of each in the US :

Central nervous system defects (brain and   spinal cord)

	1 in	total
Anencephaly (microcephaly)	4,859	859
Spina bifida without anencephaly	2,858	1,460
Encephalocele (cranial fistula)	12,235	341

Eye defects

Anophthalmia/microphthalmia	5,349	780

Cardiovascular defects (heart)

	1 in	total
Common Truncus	13,876	301
Transposition of great arteries	3,333	1,252
Tetralogy of Fallot	2,518	1,657
Atrioventricular septal defect	2,122	1,966
Hypoplastic left heart syndrome	4,344	960

Orofacial defects (middle of the face)

Cleft palate without cleft lip	1,574	2,651
Cleft lip with or without cleft palate	940	4,437

Gastrointestinal defects (esophagus, stomach, and intestines)

Esophageal atresia/tracheoesophageal fistula (narrow/disconnected windpipe)	4,608	905
Large intestine narrow/disconnected	2,138	1,952

Musculoskeletal defects (muscles and bones)

Reduction deformity, upper limbs	2,869	1,454
Reduction deformity, lower limbs	5,949	701
Gastroschisis (hole in abdomen)	2,229	1,871
Omphalocele (guts outside belly)	5,386	775
Diaphragmatic hernia (hole in diaphragm)	3,836	1,088

Chromosomal anomalies (extra chromosomes)

Trisomy 13 (multiple defects)	7,906	528
Trisomy 18 (interrupts development)	3,762	1,109
Trisomy 21 (Down syndrome)	691	6,037

("Centers for Disease Control and Prevention", 2015)[31]

1 in 33 babies born presents with a birth defect. This does not include low birth weight infants who require special intervention, a separate issue with various causes, though there is disagreement on whether it should or shouldn't be included. You are less likely to hit a roulette number with its 38 spaces, 37 if you are with James Bond on the French Riviera, than you are to have a child with a birth defect.

Those are the cold, objective odds regards birth defects. Another set of hard facts are the bills that come due with pregnancy. In the United States, carrying and birthing a child is immorally expensive, as is so much of the US health care system. And, no, it is not the best in the world.

The slightly more than 4 million births each year in the United States costs about 50 billion dollars for healthy, uncomplicated births. Depending on which region of the country you are in, cost vary. In fact, costs between hospitals in the same city can vary dramatically. Most mothers walk into prenatal and delivery costs blind and that is generally by design, a system of opaque pricing. When was the last time you saw a billboard or TV ad touting the price of an uncomplicated vaginal delivery? It is likely you could call your local hospital and ask for a price and they would not be able to, or not want to, to give you a price.

Even when researching average costs of hospital delivery alone, the figures expressed as a US average are all over the map. Digging deep, I found that each report used a variety of criteria that may have counted only what insurers paid versus what hospitals would charge. Others reached their totals by comparing paid insured costs, out of pocket patient costs and rates charged to those without insurance. Further, many hospitals tack on fees not medically related to a hospital stay and some of the reports excluded or included those fees. I think the most accurate tally would be one based on the number that arrives in the mail as a bill.

The Agency for Healthcare Research's Quality Healthcare Cost and Utilization Project produces figures that appear to be fair and reasonable. They cite an uncomplicated vaginal delivery as costing $2,900 and a complicated C-section as costing $6,800 per stay in 2008. (Podulka, 2011)[31] Beyond that, none of the other papers and reports I dug up were remotely close to the H-CUP figures cited above.

Out of the more than 20 sources I checked, I chose MappingHealth.com's figures as being the median figures on delivery costs. They cite the average C-section as being $13,061 and a vaginal delivery as $8,435. Many of the other sources I reviewed were as much as 2-6 times higher and were not able to explain discrepancies with other source figures. MappingHealth.com also compares US delivery cost to those of four other nations and the comparisons can only leave a US consumer of health delivery services depressed. Australia comes in at $9,012 and $4,052 for a C-section and vaginal delivery. France at $4,736 and $3,768; Spain at $2,989 and $2,266; Argentina at $959 and

$737. ("Mapping Health: Mapping Maternity Care and Birth Outcomes", 2016)[32] Per the Canadian Institute for Health Information, Canada comes in at $1,492 and $795 for simple C-section or vaginal delivery, just to let you know if you weren't quite depressed enough already. ("Giving Birth in Canada", 2006)[33]

The costs for a baby born with a major birth defect varies on the type of defect, severity of the defect and chosen treatment plan. These defects fall into basically two categories of either being correctable or disabling. Correctable is a onetime treatment or fix while disabling involves ongoing care for the lifetime of the child. The number of variables complicates each situation but in general correctable conditions can range from about $100,000 to $250,000 per case while costs per disabled case can run between $100,000 to $500,000 per case. In the most serious of cases with no holds barred, it is not uncommon to see lifetime costs in the millions of dollars for a permanently disabled person. The aforementioned figures are based on 1995 figures and have not been adjusted for inflation. Doubling to tripling them would be a fair estimation of 2016 costs based on annual healthcare inflation rate between 4-9%. (Californian Birth Defects Monitoring Program, 1995)[34] Other figures thrown around show that it is not atypical for a disabled child to cost 10-15 times more to raise than a healthy child.

As you can see from the aforementioned, there is a strong incentive for mothers-to-be to avoid behaviors detrimental to a developing child. Smoking, alcohol to excess, drug use licit or illicit and diet are factors generally in control of any mother to be, barring addiction or poverty. The emotional costs are extremely high and parents of a disabled child experience high levels of stress, anxiety and other personal and social dysfunctions. Many families with a seriously disabled child end up operating on the periphery of extended family and often are subjected to humiliating judgments, especially as regards finances or the child's behavior. Introducing a seriously disabled child into a social situation is fraught with risk in that people can react in wildly varying ways that make such an action an anxious endeavor, enough so that many families learn to associate only with groups that share the same challenge of a disabled child.

With Zika working its way up and into the United States, it will be take time before we know the extent of damage the virus will wreak upon the US healthcare system. Even if there is a worst case scenario of vector mosquito populations capable of transmitting the Zika virus, we will not have a full grasp well into 2017. To be certain, we should have strong clues of how hit or miss the whole situation is by early 2017 and even by the fall of 2016 as entomologists and infectious disease researchers sample the mosquito populations and test for the virus.

While certain behaviors of the mother can be controlled by her, other factors are not, be it random genetic and chromosomal problems or random environmental exposures. Short of an expectant mother locking herself in a box, there is no reasonable way to create a zero risk environment absent of mosquitoes. We all go outside for reasons necessary and healthy and it is at those times we are in the mosquito's habitat. Windows and doors of homes open and close many times in a day and most of us at one time or another have had to deal with the droning buzz of a bothersome mosquito as we tried to get to sleep.

What the Zika virus throws at us is all sorts of poor choices. For any women who wants to become pregnant, there is a host of questions they should answer prior to becoming pregnant as to what risks they are willing to take and what outcomes they will be able to tolerate. Financially alone, the costs of a major birth defect is life destructive unless you have access to a profound amount of funds. Per the US Bureau of the Census, in 2014 the average US household income pegged in at $53,500 gross, and that out-of-pocket healthcare expenses, the latest safety valve attempt to hold the line on premiums, continue to rise in order for the private insurance market to make profit and keep their product affordable to employers and individuals. Even insured persons of modest means are finding that out of pocket expenses are so onerous that they find themselves financially damaged. As health care inflation continues to be double and triple the national Consumer Price Index rate of inflation, health costs are going to continue to chew away income. It is unsustainable even with government subsidies for lower income people to purchase health insurance. It should be a serious warning sign that so many middle class people and employers are now at the point that they need serious tax dollars to   provide health plans that are becoming more and more of a dubious insurance against financial ruin. The Affordable Care Act is most likely only a temporary measure to keep the rate of uninsured down as the math is just too ugly and indisputable to pretend otherwise as medical inflation mauls the market.

For an infant born with microcephaly the costs in the US healthcare system will be astronomical. The fact that many such children can live for several decades is the bulk of the total cost. While some microcephalics are able to achieve some level of function, and that even about 10% become somewhat functionally independent, the rest are dependent for life and deal with numerous maladies involving the other major organ systems. Most suffer major mobility problems. Fine motor control is limited to nonexistent. In very rare cases, such children may learn to speak and even read. The vast majority suffer major cognitive deficits. Of course, there is a wide swath of variability but none of that variability completely ameliorates the personal and social burdens on child and family.

Further complicating matters is that 40% of pregnancies

are unintended, meaning the mother may not know she is pregnant until the 5-8 weeks after conception. It's difficult to take proactive measures to support a healthy pregnancy when you aren't aware you are pregnant, let alone make preparations for being outdoors exposed to a bug we've been conditioned to believe over a lifetime is nothing more than minor nuisance, not a possible life altering encounter. For persons raised in rattlesnake country, they take precautions while outdoors that are second nature to how they interact with the environment. It will be getting us to change our behavior regards the mosquito that is going to be the greatest challenge. We will have to think differently on a range of activities of daily living from property maintenance to social gatherings to whether or not to attend outdoor summer celebrations. I'm not so certain that such changes will be at the forefront of our thinking as we go about our busy lives.

Matters of Conscience

Here's what we know so far: 1) The United States population is virgin to Zika; 2) Two types of mosquito are capable vectors and together they are common in one third of the country, that being the South up into the Ohio valley and somewhat north of that yet plus about 100-200 miles west of the Mississippi River. Within that area about 150 million Americans reside; 3) Microcephaly and Guillain-Barre are appearing in dramatic jumps over normal occurrences in areas infected with Zika in Latin America; 4) The Zika virus has been found to be present by testing and verbal patient history in gestating mothers and those who have given birth to microcephalic children; 5) A child with a major birth defect is a serious complication to the parent's emotional, social and financial health.

The known is that women who become pregnant and then become infected with Zika during that pregnancy, especially in the first trimester, risk giving birth to a seriously ill infant. We also know that in the United States that about 40% of pregnancies are unintended and that most mothers do not have knowledge of their own pregnancy until about 6-8 weeks after conception, creating a serious problem of ignorance that may contribute to an increased risk of an unhealthy gestation. As testing for the virus stands now, there is only a 2-7 day window where there is enough of a detectable viral load and that testing is unlikely to happen since 75% of Zika infections are asymptomatic. Who goes to the doctor for testing of a possible infectious agent when they are feeling well? Pretty much no one.

We know there are 6 million pregnancies annually within the United States. Running on assumption with back of the envelope calculations, we can figure that about half those pregnancies will happen where half the US population resides, that is in the eastern third of the United States. This leaves us with about 3 million possible pregnancies in *A. aegypti* and *A. albopictus* habitat.

Of the 3 million pregnancies, 40% will be unplanned, leaving a number of 1.2 million women who will have no idea, nor plan, they are or could be pregnant until about 6-8 weeks into the gestation. Currently, the US odds of having a microcephalic baby are 1 in 4,859, meaning that out 1.2 million unintended pregnancies there would be a total of 246 with microcephaly absent any influence of Zika. Obviously, intended or unintended, microcephaly will occur. I make the distinction because with intended pregnancies mothers have some protection by being able to make conscientious efforts at prevention, even though such prevention efforts do not provide total protection from having a child with a birth defect.

Brazil is removing some of the guess work from the odds. In 2014, Brazil reported 150 cases of microcephaly nationwide. 2015 is revealing a figure of 270 confirmed cases per the latest tallies coming out of the Brazilian Ministry of Health. Frankly, about all that should elicit is a big fat shrug of the shoulders.

The Cytomegalo virus (CMV) actually makes for a good comparison and reality check: When pregnant women catch CMV, only about 35% transmit the virus to the developing fetus. Out of those 35% of fetuses that become infected, approximately 20% are born with a major birth defect. The final numbers end up being that a baby who developed when the mother was infected with CMV has only a 1 in 15 chance of suffering permanent harm. With something as devastating as CMV, 'only 1 of 15' is an unacceptable odd. CMV is responsible for a total of around 5,000 permanently disabled children being born each year per the CDC's latest count in 2013.

However, what makes CMV less frightening is that it is a known quantity, the US population is no longer immunologically naïve and over 70% of people in the developed world have been exposed and are now generally immune. The risk is to those who are not immune, thus it is imperative that women trying to get pregnant or who are pregnant need to pay high attention to personal hygiene especially as regards being around children, touching their toys, changing diapers or any other way urine, feces and saliva travels by way of child.

Now that we have some context regards the Zika virus by way of comparison with other birth defects, and that we know there is a 1 in 33 chance of having a child with a major birth defect, what are the mother's options? In the case of the introduction of a new risk that is foreseeable but still has many unanswered questions, especially regards the odds and whether or not there is a true and direct link, great uncertainty is created.

The first question a woman of child bearing age needs to answer for herself is what her risk profile is, that is, does she live in an area where the two types of mosquito are present. The greater risks of a having a child with a birth defect are maternal behaviors of smoking, substance abuse nutritional quality and environmental exposures ranging from bacterial and viral to chemical. Genetic issues are usually unknown and thus can't factor into a decision.

Birth control is a preventive measure that greatly reduces the risk of a birth defect pregnancy. It is access to birth control that is part of a women's risk profile for unintended pregnancy. We know that in more rural areas where medical access is limited and difficult to get to, rates of unintended pregnancies are higher. Also, women with limited purchasing power are also more likely to have accidental pregnancies. We are seeing in Texas counties that where women's health clinics that once provided affordable or free contraceptives and are now shut down, that the number of pregnancies has shot up by noticeable amounts. (Stevenson, "New England Journal of Medicine")[34] The Stevenson et al study discovered that the numbers of women accessing long-acting birth control measures such as levonorgestrel, which is placed under the skin, intrauterine devices or contraceptive injections from state supported family planning services, dropped by about a third after Planned Parenthood was kicked out of family planning programs. Meanwhile, low-income women who had previously been receiving injectable contraceptives from Planned Parenthood before the change saw their birth rate shoot up 27 percent.

In a Washington Post interview, the lead author of the study, Joseph Potter, is explicit that it is possible that the women merely decided to get pregnant or went elsewhere to get contraception. Without interviewing each and every mother, such a possibility has to be admitted. This admission is now being hammered by Texas politicians who have been openly hostile to Planned Parenthood and in 2013 guaranteed that the loss of Planned Parenthood clinics, or PP's loss of ability to distribute contraceptives, would have zero effect on pregnancy rates. The Washington Post further writes that Rick Allgeyer, a research director at the Texas Health and Human Services Commission, had worked in conjunction with researchers from University of Texas--Austin's Population Research Center to examine what had happened after Texas cut off Planned Parenthood funding and inclusion from its government sponsored Women's Health Program in 2013. Some Texas pols consider Allgeyer's work to be outside of his job description, though to most observers, it appears such a study fits entirely under his job description. Allgeyer has since quit. (Kaplan, 2016)[35]

The Texas officials who in 2013 promised there would be no change in access to contraceptives or in pregnancy rates just had their rear ends handed to them on a gold platter, that gold platter being the New England Journal of Medicine which has a pretty solid reputation for not catering to cranks and demanding rigorous compliance by way of editorial board and peer review processes. About the most apt analogy I can make is the NEJM is the NASA of medical journals. These are intelligent people whose biggest fear in life is looking stupid, something that cannot be said about more than few opponents of family planning. One such person hardly bothered by facts is Texas Senator Jane Nelson, builder of the 2013 Women's Health Program, a program title intentionally crafted to mislead people to believe the program was about improving women's health when in fact it attacks women's health. With the NEJM publication of findings regards the uptick in certain Texas county pregnancies, especially in light of Nelson's and her co-conspirators outright denial of the data presented, they look foolish—and by any objective measure or a sympathetic one, 'foolish' is being charitable.

Any time a tool or item is made easier to access, the more times that item will be used. If we removed every screw driver from every house in America, the number of screws turned per year would drop dramatically. If we put a handgun on every dinner table in every household in America, shootings would go up simply due to ease of access and availability. If you throw down 10,000 nails on your driveway, you're likely to get a flat tire. If you have no nails on your driveway, you'll never get a flat tire from a nail in your driveway. It stands to reason that the 27% uptick in pregnancies in the Texas counties where PP was booted is due in large part to lack of access to birth control, which is

PP's primary mission.

Texas has decided as a matter of public policy that its women should face increased risks of delivering a birth defect afflicted child. Texas officials believe that the women of childbearing age should reflect the state position that all pregnancies are valuable and that no one should interfere with any pregnancy, including the mother and in spite of any possible increased risks to her health. And, yes, every pregnancy poses an increase in risk to any mother's health, be it acute or chronic with about 90% of post partum women reporting at least one health problem with 31% reporting continuing problem(s) 6 months out. Per WHO, 297,000 maternal deaths occurred in 2013 directly related pregnancy. (GBD 2013 Mortality and Causes of Death Collaborators, 2014)[36]

Health problems can range from the expected and minor such as acute bouts of morning sickness and ankle swelling to moderate post partum chronic issues like back pain and urinary bladder dysfunction to gestational event life threatening blood clotting, placental rupture and massive hemorrhage plus multiple other conditions simply too numerous to list here.

Matters of conscience are also matters of politics, which is about the worst arena for a thoughtful, considered discussion of personal health issues simply because too often politics has proven itself to have little problem ignoring facts and evidence that do not support a position. Women of child bearing age are treated by certain leaders as if they're all bimbos or callous harpies that like to stick sharp sticks in the eyes of puppies, that their biological standing revokes various civil liberties most of us take for granted, namely that we can conduct our treatment plans as we see fit in line with our desires, needs or abilities. It simply is not rational to declare an unborn child as having rights equal to the mother than demand the mother bare disproportionate risk. Generally, respect for bodily autonomy and integrity extends even to death in that once a person passes, they, or someone acting in their stead as designated guardian, does not have to surrender so much as an eyelash for research department or organ bank. However, with pregnant women, respect for bodily autonomy is in short supply in many political and religious arenas.

I could pick on Texas some more but that would be narrow. Go back to Chapter 2 "The Mosquito" and look at the map of *Aedes aegypti's* range. The primary range for our Zika carrying little friend in the US is Texas, Louisiana, Mississippi, Alabama, Georgia and Florida, traditional pockets of political power that are hostile to women's rights and public safety net programs. The hostility bends so far as to force pregnant women to undergo waiting periods or view certain items like fetal ultrasounds, usually in the name of informed consent. Informed decisions are wonderful but, oddly, the same concern for informed consent doesn't seem to extend to information being medically accurate or encompassing, allowing some groups to deliberately pose as medically competent in order to deliberately mislead women about all their options. Further, induced abortion is the only medical procedure within the United States where states are putting waiting periods into place and the only medical procedure where certain groups are allowed, even encouraged, to disseminate information based more on religious or political values than accurate science.

One such recent case is the Purdue Students for Life campaign of February, 2016 that targeted black women with a poster campaign of "Hands Up! Don't Abort!", mimicking the Black Lives Matter movement concerned over police shootings of unarmed African-Americans. When Purdue Students for Life were probed about their campaign, they claimed that abortion providers were part of an ongoing covert campaign by white Americans to wipe out the black race. Of course, such a poster campaign by

PSL and other like groups is an effort to capitalize on suspicion and mistrust created within the black community by our country's entirely real history of slavery and Jim Crow. PSL and other like groups are fond of pointing out that minority women have a higher per capita rate of abortion than whites. That is true. However, about 69% of pregnancies amongst African-Americans are unintended vs about 40% for whites. Further, communities of color in general have higher rates of economic insecurity. I see no big mystery as to why the per capita rate of abortion would be higher amongst African-Americans. Also, such groups posit that medical abortions carry a high risk of death by including illegal abortions from countries where the procedure is a criminal act. However, in countries where it is legal, the death rate is about 0.6 per 100,000 procedures, making it safer than taking an antibiotic. ("Abortion Statistics, Facts About Abortion In The US.")[37]

Oddly enough, the rest of the medical community gets off the hook when one considers that surgeons and other physicians are in a position of power over the helpless to knock off people at will with botched surgeries or toxic prescription drugs, or merely by refusing to provide treatment. If risk reduction was the true goal, anesthesiologists and plastic surgeons would be at the head of the line for tighter restrictions.

Kansas and Oklahoma have passed laws outlawing Dilation and Extraction procedures on pregnant women who choose to abort. D&E is normally performed after 14 weeks as it is safer and more comfortable than medical induction since medical induction involves putting the mother into premature labor through the use of a variety drugs and can take days to complete if it is done after 14 weeks. Often times post 14 week induction may require a hospital stay but D&E is entirely outpatient. So what Kansas and Oklahoma have done is essentially forced physicians to abandon a known, safer technique for a mandatory less safe procedure. Both states in this instance couldn't care less about the patient and in fact purposely created a riskier situation in order to intimidate patients from making the choice to end a pregnancy. The response of some of the politicians leading the charge is they have strongly insinuated that abortion providers preferred D&E for financial gain or deliberately advocated for D&E to put their patient's lives at risk. Of course, not a lick of evidence has ever been presented to back up such claims and it defies reason and intelligence that any doctor would deliberately engage in higher risk procedures as a means to express contempt or invite scrutiny of injured or dead outcomes. The current death rate in the US for safe abortion is about 0.6 per 100,000 while WHO estimates the death rate from unsafe abortion is approximately 68,000 annually where abortion is illegal, putting the risk ratio at 1 per 270. ("Wikipedia", 2015)[38]

With the coming wave of Zika virus riding into the United States, there will be too many women who have to make decisions on how they wish to proceed with family planning. If Brazil is any indication of what we can expect, it is going to get chaotic. Already in Brazil and several other Latin American countries, Women on the Web reports it is seeing a dramatic increase in requests for Mifepristone and Misoprostol, two drugs used to induce miscarriage during the first trimester.

According to the Davis Drug Guide, Mifepristone, RU-486, is a synthetic steroid designed to bind to the intracellular progesterone receptor, blocking the effects of progesterone. When used for the termination of pregnancy, this leads to contractions that triggers activity in the myometrium, the middle layer of the uterine wall, and causes the uterus to shed the placenta and its contents. Misoprostol is given in conjunction to reduce nausea and is a medication used to induce labor and cause an abortion plus reduce postpartum bleeding due to poor contraction of the uterus.

Women on the Web (https://www.womenonweb.org) is dedicated to providing access to contraceptives pre and post conception and provides the majority of product by way of package delivery services. For those women seeking an abortion, Women on the Web states that a doctor can only help if the woman: a) lives in a country where access to safe abortion is restricted; b)she is less than 9 weeks pregnant; c)has no severe illnesses.

In Catholic Latin America, such work as done by Women on the Web is controversial. In El Salvador, all abortion for any reason is illegal while other countries make exceptions for the life of the mother or cases of rape and incest. The anxiety generated by the spread and presence of the Zika virus is alone problematic but coupled with pregnancy and the increased odds of having a child with a severe birth defect, that anxiety no doubt borders on panic for many. In a nod to reason and compassion, Pope Francis has stated that it is a lesser problem to prevent a pregnancy than to terminate a pregnancy and that in certain situations such as the Zika outbreak, contraception is an act of legitimate self defense, using the case where Pope Paul VI in the early 1960s granted a papal dispensation to nuns living in the Belgian Congo who were in grave danger of being raped to use oral contraceptives.

Women in Latin America are certainly between a rock and hard place regards pregnancy and Zika while women in the United States have more options. However, in some states those options are being whittled back, be it access to birth control or abortion services. Indiana is currently attempting to pass a law where no child may be aborted for the reason of a fetal diagnosis of a disability or gender. What is truly odd about the law is that no reason need to be given for any abortion prior to 20 weeks in Indiana. However, if it is suspected that the birthed infant would die within three months post partum, then it would be OK to go ahead and get an abortion for the reason of birth defect. Doctors tend to be fairly intelligent but I've come across exactly zero who can read minds. Additionally, the business of making prognostication on time of death, especially regards a fetus, is fairly dicey. Medically speaking, such laws are embarrassing. Yet other states have forged ahead. In 2013 North Dakota made it illegal for a doctor to perform an abortion because of fetal genetic anomalies, including Down syndrome. Indiana, Missouri and South Dakota considered or are considering similar laws this year. Seven other states-- Arizona, Kansas, North Carolina, North Dakota, Oklahoma, Pennsylvania and South Dakota, have laws banning abortions if the reason is gender selection. In 2012, the United States House of Representatives rejected such a measure. Further, Arizona's law also forbids abortion when the doctor knows that the abortion is being sought based on the sex or race of the child, or the race of a parent of that child. (Lewin, 2015)[39]

As spurious as such reasons mentioned above may or may not be for a women to choose to abort, it is impossible to enforce unless the above mentioned states have plans to start subpoenaing abortion clinic client lists and one by one conduct interrogations of the women to make such a determination.

For gestating women who discover they've become Zika infected, there is a genuine reason to believe they are at increased risk of having a messed up pregnancy that may conclude with the delivery of a profoundly ill child. For lawmakers to wag their fingers that disability as a reason to abort a pregnancy is illegal is not going to play well in those states where Zika shows up this coming summer in 2016. I have no doubt that anti choice legislators will have no problem overlooking the problematic dimensions introduced by a Zika outbreak. Most disconcerting is that many of these same anti choice lawmakers are openly hostile to safety net programs, as if pregnancy is a moral failing so the mother to be must be punished by acts of omission, inaction and denial.

How these matters of conscience play out across the United States in 2016 and beyond will be interesting. For any young woman who is attempting to become pregnant or finds herself unexpectedly pregnant where a Zika outbreak is identified, they will be forced to factor that in to any decision they make. She will have to deal with serious misinformation and experts' uncertainty since the situation continues to be highly fluid until more concrete facts are ascertained. This is a problem where the most trusted source will be those who openly and freely proclaim they do not know or that competing ideas may all have at least some validity. Gray is the only color that can describe Zika and the United States today and likely for the next one to two years, hardly the comforting guidance needed by persons who have serious choices to make.

The Plan

The Plan is that there is no plan. While WHO and PAHO have declared an international emergency, more than a few experts think that WHO might be a little gun shy due to the criticism they received in their initial tepid response to the West Africa Ebola crisis, the result being an overly sensitive response to the Zika outbreak. My reaction to that is that with 7 billion people on the planet, there will always be enough people to have a different view of matters to make their voices heard. As of now, WHO and PAHO are perfectly within reason to sound the alarm. One measure of how serious a crisis is, is to see how much effort is going into attacking, covering up or denying it exists.

Brazil has the military out on the streets with something close to 250,000 soldiers and volunteers spraying larvicide in hopes of tamping down the mosquito population to at least project an appearance of a dedicated effort to keeping the expected crowds safe for the Rio Olympics. If their intensity of the effort to eradicate mosquito breeding habitat continues up to and through the games in August, they should have things well under control. However, in a nation the size of Brazil, 3.3 million sq miles vs 3.7 US total, rural areas will likely receive little benefit from such efforts but that remains to be seen.

Venezuela appears to be taking the opposite tact of Brazil's aggressive efforts. The official line coming out of Venezuela's Health Ministry is no line at all. In 2015 they began withholding all sorts of medical data, including infectious disease reports. Thus far, the best measure of how large the Zika outbreak is in Venezuela is coming from neighboring Columbia where the shared border has thousands from both countries crossing the border every day for work or family reasons. In many places, the border is unsecured and not monitored, meaning that if a infectious disease health crisis more contagious than Zika were to break out, an important screening tool of health checks at border stations is absent. Colombian officials guestimate the number of Zika infections at around 400,000 based on how many Venezuelans they've treated in their hospitals. ("Firstpost Venezuela doctors fume.... Zika cases", 2016)[40]

Aggravating Venezuela's problems is the utter incompetence of how they've managed their economy through a series of price controls that force local purchasers of foreign product to eliminate the costs of raw materials as part of the retail price. If a loaf of bread in Canada rises from $1 to $2, a Venezuelan importer of Canadian bread pays the increased price but he is not allowed to pass it on to his customers via a higher retail price. Price controls remove the agility needed for businesses to adjust to changing economics and in Venezuela's case, it has forced many businesses to shutter. This situation has trickled into the health care system and normally reliable suppliers of medical supplies and equipment are unable to supply product except at a loss. I think of Venezuela's condition as the socialist version of the crackpot economic theory the Laffer Curve where the fairy tale belief is that the further you cut taxes the more government revenue increases, both cases stupefyingly out of touch with the realities of math. In the meantime, a potentially catastrophic situation is simply pretended to not exist in Venezuela.

You don't need incompetent government to screw up an already wonderful crisis. Citizens are remarkably adept at insulating themselves from bad news by believing any number of rationalizations ranging from believing they are a good person to conspiracy theories that such events are propaganda attempts to control the population for nefarious goals. Naturally, the same types of thinking bleed into the elected governments as well and I strongly suspect certain US states will downplay the Zika issue.

Texas, where *A. aegypti* thrives, especially in the more moist, humid eastern portion of the state, is poised to be in the thick of any Zika outbreak. As of this writing, there appears to be a collective shrug going on at the Texas Department of State Health Services. Granted, their primary mission is not mosquito control since that is generally delegated a county and municipal concern. Some counties such as Dallas County are stepping up monitoring efforts with plans for more diligent mosquito habitat control while others have expressed that they feel their current programs are adequate. At this time, what is missing is a top down management plan that transcends civil borders and can be a loci of information, organization and resource sharing.

The United States is often accused of having a short memory. When the Ebola crisis reared up in 2014, the federal Center for Disease Control and Protection offered advice and some testing assistance to hospitals as well as state and local health departments on how to handle a suspected or confirmed case of Ebola. When Dallas Presbyterian had an Ebola positive patient come through their doors, a Liberian national visiting relatives in Dallas, they muffed it by first missing the fact the patient haled from an Ebola crisis region and chalking up his feverish symptoms as the flu. Several days later, the poor man returned and this time his nationality and port of egress triggered inquiry that led to his Ebola diagnosis. What compounded the original error was the staff assigned to the patient had less than adequate training, biohazard protective gear and decontamination procedures. The result was two infected staff who then went out and about in the community, with one going so far as to travel by commercial air to Ohio. Fortunately, nothing came of this misstep but the CDC was roundly criticized for leaving state and local health departments to fashion their own response plans. After the Dallas incident, the CDC did become more involved and took a more firm lead in organizing training and response.

As of now, the CDC has issued guidelines to health professionals that recommend who should be tested for Zika: Mothers who report having traveled to or are in a known Zika infected area; Zika should be suspected in an infant or child under 18 years old that traveled to, or lived in, an affected area within the past 2 weeks; or has two or more of the following signs/symptoms: fever, rash, conjunctivitis, or arthralgia. Any positive results need to be reported to local or state authorities because Zika is a nationally notifiable condition. The CDC update goes on to suggest that ultrasounds be done in the 2nd trimester along with routine prenatal cares. Other information advises how to test for Zika, such as cerebral spinal fluid sampling and that if a child is born with microcephaly, or the mother was positive or inconclusive for Zika, the baby should be tested. Also, doctors should rule out leptospirosis, malaria, rickettsia, group A streptococcus, rubella, measles, and parvovirus, enterovirus, adenovirus, and alphavirus infections. The line that sums up the 'Good Luck' plan is, "Local health officials will need to determine when to implement testing recommendations for pregnant women without symptoms based on information about local levels of Zika virus transmission and local laboratory capacity." (Texas DSHS, "– Health Care Professionals", 2016)[41]

As plans go, it can be summed up this way: Try not to get mosquito bit; that your doctor should look for Zika if there are signs or symptoms of Zika, or the mother has been to or is an area where there is an active Zika outbreak.

I am not inspired. Nor should you be.

Mosquito control efforts are all being left to local governments to decide what to do based on vector control methods already in place for existing mosquito control with the only additional new item being that trapped *A. aegypti* and *A. albopictus* mosquitoes be tested for the presence of Zika.

Again, there is no overarching umbrella agency or revised or new chain of command to monitor or issue direction or coordinate action as is usually needed or beneficial during a public emergency. If there was a single lesson learned out of the disaster of Hurricane Katrina it was that an actionable organization that could receive and send information and resources, plus be the final authority transcending civil borders, was imperative and essential. We do not have that with Zika. It is trying and nerve wracking enough for emergency personnel to have had training runs dealing with possible future emergencies that even when the real thing happens it still is a crisis that is difficult to manage. Even though the CDC has activated its Emergency Response Operations to work with the American Academy of Pediatricians to better distribute testing and treatment guidelines, there has been little done to marshal resources for mosquito control and safety net programs. If Zika blows up in our faces across the southern states this summer or next, we don't even have the skeleton of an algorithm in place to guide us towards the same page. About the only good thing one can conclude is that there is no recipe for disaster because there isn't even a recipe.

Realistically, about all doctors can do is react to what appears in their offices and urge women of child bearing age to go or stay on contraceptives and use mosquito repellant. Where the real battle will be is with the local mosquito control folks, about as an anonymous work force as there possibly is if my personal knowledge is any sort of accurate guide. Once a person is infected, there isn't anything that can be done other than gather as much information as possible as time unfolds and see if a problem has developed. No doubt the ultrasound machines will be working overtime in the coming months and that every fetal head noted to be smaller than normal will trigger all sorts of anxiety.

Even though we have this huge heads up about a very real impending health disaster, there is a lot of 'wait and see' being exhibited in official pronouncements. Yes, the precautions are being published but overall there is no sense of genuine urgency. To be charitable, would it do anyone any good to get all riled up at this time? Probably not. But it wouldn't hurt to start getting an interstate Plan of Action into place to identify trouble spots and assist the have-nots with adequate funds as needed for prevention efforts.

On the Texas border of the Rio Grande, many of the counties have pockets of migrant workers encamped into shanty towns that are every bit as third world as other places on the globe, complete with poor sanitation, standing water and untended refuse ranging from discarded tires to simple garbage like soda cups that become mosquito egg incubators. Many of these counties have budgets that hang on by a thread from year to year, their state funding and assistance more tenuous and lacking as tax hating politicians slash into the meat and bone of critical public services. Even when it is demonstrated that a policy has had negative outcomes, such as the slashing of family planning clinic budgets and the increased rise in pregnancies, the response was to fire the messenger, bury their heads in the sand and stomp their feet that the bad news was all a plot.

Again, I appear to be picking on poor ol' Texas. You may insert the names of all the Gulf of Mexico states plus Georgia, South Carolina and Oklahoma in place of Texas. Not one of the states aforementioned is putting together a plan on the state level for a coordinated response should the wave of an epidemic break. A review of the various aforementioned state websites shows only Florida to have taken the matter seriously enough to declare a state health emergency in four counties and ordered an increase in efforts towards mosquito control. Louisiana has enough problems with projected budget shortfalls that it appears to be relying on current mosquito control methods, though to their credit they are finally taking the Medicaid expansion offered by the 2009 Affordable Care Act. Georgia dedicates a minor web page of Q&A about Zika covering prevention measures and travel advice. Alabama has issued travel and mosquito control advisories with Mississippi doing the same. Oklahoma and South Carolina make minor mention with no discernible plan executed on a state level. As it stands, what plans exist are decidedly reactionary and that any person who has the misfortune to somehow be affected by the Zika virus they will be on their own, empowered only to the extent of their personal resources and health plans.

From this side of the coming wave, the dollars and cents of a potential emergency is that doing nothing is cheaper than over prepping and not having to execute, tying up or wasting dollars that could be dedicated to more defined needs. This may be a case of penny wise and pound foolish or it may be a national expression of 'Your problem. Good luck' that pervades a part of our political spectrum. We have been given a chance to roll the dice and have decidedly chosen to gamble.

As of February 19, 2016 a WHO situation report attempts to demonstrate a corollary case for increased incidents of Guillain-Barre and microcephaly where the Zika outbreak has been measurable. Reducing it to odds at this point is a squishy business but the trend is clear: cases of microcephaly and G-B have increased 4 to 10 fold depending on the area reporting.

On February 18, 2016, WHO issued a Situation Report to the general media that the World Bank Group announced that it had made $150 million US immediately available to support countries in Latin America and the Caribbean affected by the Zika virus outbreak. This amount follows the WHO declaration of a Public Health Emergency of International Concern (PHEIC)on February 1, 2016 for the recent cluster of microcephaly cases and other neurological disorders reported in the Americas amid the growing Zika virus outbreak. The World Bank Group has engaged with governments across the region, including sending technical experts to affected countries. If additional financing is needed, the World Bank Group stands ready to increase its support. On an international effort, a strategy is being produced with a backbone of funding. The US itself is not as organized and thus far shows very spotty effort.

Back of the envelope figuring shows that the United States can expect about 4 million Zika infections in 2016 and 2017 with the majority of those likely confined to the Gulf of Mexico states, *A. aegypti's* primary range in the United States. If cases of microcephaly and G-B follow a similar pattern as they have thus far in Latin America, the United States should see similar results.

The current rate of G-B is 1/100,000 in the US. Texas, Louisiana, Alabama, Mississippi and Florida have a combined population of about 58 million per US Census Bureau Quick Facts. That would be 580 cases of G-B under usual circumstances. The incidence of microcephaly is 1 in 4859 births. Total 2013 birth rate for Texas,

Louisiana, Alabama, Mississippi and Florida was about 762,000 with 156 reported cases of microcephaly. Using the conservative end of ratios coming out of Latin America showing the 4-10 fold increase in G-B and microcephaly, that would yield 624 cases of microcephaly and 2,320 cases of G-B in those five states. A high estimate would put this at 5,800 G-B cases and 1,560 microcephaly cases. I have to caution that these numbers are highly fluid and based on all things being considered equal between Latin America and the United States. That's a lot of room for 'ifs' and 'maybes'.

The total number of new cases in our five Gulf Coast states shows a conservative total of extra cases due to Zika to be roughly 2,208 for both G-B and microcephaly. At a low ball dollar figure of $100,000 for medical care per case that comes in at an additional $220,800,000 annually. A high end figure would be about $1,140,000,000 amongst 5 states. Again, good odds are difficult to come by due to the fluid nature of the current crisis, varying billing charges between hospitals and the completeness of data being collected. The longer the Zika epidemic lasts the more clear we'll see things. Keep in mind that we haven't even considered the remaining states extending up just north of the Ohio Valley and several hundred miles west of the Mississippi River where *A. albopictus* is commonly found. Also, by my own admission, the $100,000 figure would be considered laughably low by many experts, especially since a microcephalic baby so often has so many other comorbidities and long term care needs beyond the first year. It is easy to make a case for 5-15 billion dollars in direct costs to a moderate Zika outbreak affecting 4 million people.

In light of our back of the envelope figures, it's much easier to start getting motivated about having a plan and getting to know those in charge of mosquito control efforts which, not surprisingly, is easier said than done. Mosquito control budgets are set a variety ways but most states provide an annual line item divvied amongst various mosquito control districts supplemented with local funding. However, such local discretion creates a patchwork of effort and results. One township, parish or city may value mosquito control more than another, making serious efforts to ensure proper funding to achieve desired suppression levels. Other government entities may view mosquito suppression efforts as a discretionary expense standing in line behind other commitments or wants. Louisiana and Florida have highly organized networks of mosquito districts while more northern states like Illinois and Indiana that deal with *A. albopictus* rather than *A. aegypti* have control efforts that are spotty with little state oversight.

Typical mosquito control measures involve killing the mosquito, killing the larvae or destroying the eggs. Sprays and traps can both be used. An ovitrap is designed to be an attractive option for mosquito egg laying and can be placed just about anywhere. The trap is laced with either an adulticide or larvicide to kill the adult mosquito or its eggs. Often times both are used together. The traps have the added benefit of making it easy to see the types of mosquitoes that are in an area and to test them for various diseases. Also, these traps can be used with or without spraying and for more targeted problem areas.

Communities that seek to control adult mosquitoes to combat an outbreak of mosquito-borne disease or a very heavy nuisance infestation of mosquitoes will use EPA registered pesticides known as adulticides. They are applied either by aircraft or by ground with trucks outfitted with sprayers. State and local governments commonly use the organophosphate insecticides like malathion and naled or the synthetic pyrethroid insecticides prallethrin, etofenprox, pyrethrins, permethrin, resmethrin and sumithrin for adult mosquito control. ("EPA", 2016)[42]

Mosquito adulticides are applied as ultra-low volume

(ULV) sprays, able to do so since ULV sprayers eject a very fine mist curtain of droplets so light that they remain airborne and kill flying mosquitoes when there is contact. ULV applications employ small quantities of a chemically active ingredient in relation to the size of the area treated, typically less than 80 grams (about 3 ounces) per acre. This is done to reduce exposure risk to sensitive people and environments and control costs.

Many people have suspicions of chemicals, especially those used on a large scale in agriculture or other venues. Mosquito larvicide and adulticide can be used for large scale mosquito control programs without posing risks of concern to the general population or to the environment when used as instructed. An example of a chemical that has raised general public wariness is DDT. DDT (dichlorodiphenyltrichloroethane) is an excellent insecticide but its widespread use was famously questioned in Rachel Carson's 1962 book *"Silent Spring"*. Many people believe that DDT has been outright banned. That is false. It is tightly restricted and regulated and its use, or lack of use, remains controversial since DDT had proven itself to be an excellent mosquito control tool to prevent mosquito borne infections, especially malaria. Use of DDT in the United States is restricted to tight permitting only in cases of agricultural or human emergency.

What made DDT so controversial was the discovery that DDT is an endocrine disruptor which can cause problems during gestation leading to premature birth or miscarriage in mammals. DDT was also pinned for being liable for the thin egg shells that could not withstand normal incubation pressures. The American Bald Eagle and DDT are practically mentioned in the same sentence since so many of us associate the bald eagle's former endangered species status and wonderful comeback with the use and near-ban on DDT. So, yes, it's with good reason we question the widespread use and applications of various '-cides'.

Will local and state governments rise to meet Zika and stop it in its tracks by taking preventive measures that include upgraded, refined pesticide spraying and other methods? Thus far, there is little noise being made other than relatively anonymous education campaigns that appear to be confined to state or federal agency websites like the EPA, CDC or NIH. Many state websites provide outline information on Zika along with links to more in-depth information on federal websites, leaving the impression they are aren't all that concerned. Whether there will be increased use of spraying or trap setting is largely being left to the individual mosquito control districts in each state or whatever other government entity is in charge of such a thing.

The other angle that is used in mosquito control is source control. Source control is the process of identifying and destroying mosquito habitat in order to prevent mosquitoes from breeding and laying. In the 19th and 20th centuries, a popular form of source control was to drain wetlands, ponds and other natural areas that contained standing water. The thinking was not only were mosquitoes being denied breeding habitat but we were taking nontillable acres and creating farm lands. We became so good at this in part by noticing and appreciating the wonderful success of reduced mosquito nuisance, further prodding us on to drain even more wetlands. Soon enough, though, we began to recognize that the destruction of once thought 'useless swamps' was really a knuckleheaded and shortsighted campaign of destruction of valuable wildlife habitat that supported sustainable and economically viable harvests of clams, oysters, waterfowl, fish and other dinner table fare. Additionally, it was found that wetlands were important water retention, water filtration and ground water recharging areas as well as critical breeding habitat for hundreds of species of bird, reptile and mammal wildlife.

Even today, after the destruction or alteration of over 90% of America's wetlands, many people continue to insist that more wetland drainage be allowed. Some things never will go extinct and shortsightedness appears to one such item that falls into that category.

Today, the source control emphasized is the spraying of certain habitat such as stagnant waters in ditches or other areas but only with limited amounts to minimize disruptions. More popular source control measures are eliminating items like cups, tires or any item that holds water where a mosquito could lay its eggs. In one sense, source control can be thought of as a trash clean up and beautification effort. No one is upset to see a pile of tires taken away for recycling or roadside ditches missing fast food trash.

The most important aspect of source control falls to private property owners to police their own yards for mosquito habitat. Bird baths, fountains, gardening water buckets or any other place or item that can hold water should have the water changed weekly to interrupt the mosquito life cycle. Spraying can be useful and can have near immediate results but the suppression of standing water has been found to be as effective over time, thus a fine excuse to spare money and pesticide exposure.

A third method of control that is controversial for all the wrong reasons is the use of genetically modified organisms, which in this case would be genetically modified mosquitoes. Oxitec, a United Kingdom company, is in the business of breeding sterile mosquitoes for release into the wild. What they have done is isolated DNA that can be inserted into mosquito eggs that is then incorporated into the mosquito's genome. They do this with hundreds of eggs in hopes of getting one that will cut and paste the inserted DNA into the genome. If a hatched mosquito is a male, a successful gene transfer will have been effected in the male's sperm. If it is a female, a successful transfer of the modifying DNA will be present in her eggs. Since a typical mosquito egg is only 1mm long, you can only imagine this is extremely delicate work and Oxitech, short for Oxford Insect Technologies, readily admits the process kills most of the eggs or the DNA doesn't take. In the end, persistence wins out and a successful gene transfer matures to adulthood where the now modified mosquito is bred to pass on the protein interrupting modified gene.

My first thought was, 'What good is a bunch of sterile mosquitoes that can't propagate?' Oxitech's GMO mosquito propagates quite well which, of course, is what you need if you want the modified gene passed on. How the gene works is that breeding and egg laying go forward as normal but the offspring have a cellular protein interrupting self-destruct gene that kicks in at about two weeks, long enough for them to pass on the self destruct gene themselves into the rest of the *A. aegypti* mosquito population. In a lab situation, a couple of weeks survival is not feasible so the GMO mosquitoes are given tetracycline, an antibiotic, to suppress the gene. Out in the wild, though, tetracycline isn't available so the autocidal modified gene does its job in killing its own host, the GMO mosquito.

GMO has detractors and they have a point. What if we introduce a gene that somehow manages to somehow be expressed in a way that is detrimental to the normal flora or fauna. How do you get those mosquitoes, or whatever modification, back? Then there is the concern that even the pesky mosquito fills a niche in the environmental tapestry and that altering its population densities could be disruptive to other species. Most scientists think that the hundreds of other types of mosquitoes that don't bother humans will easily fill that niche so there should be no problem. I could write another book on such hypothetical situations but for now I'd have to go with the plan that has shown positive results since 2012, and that is the 80% plus reduction where Oxitech has released their GMO *A. aegypti* mosquitoes. To get rid of the Zika virus, you have to get rid of the mosquito that carries it. (Specter, "The New Yorker")[43]

I can predict with amazing accuracy that when the use and introduction of GMO mosquitoes as part of a plan to control Zika is bought up somewhere in the US, there will be vociferous protests against its use. There shouldn't be. One idiotic rumor floating around the internet is that it is a GMO mosquito responsible for the Zika outbreak in Brazil, an amazing feat since that where Zika is present the nearest GMO mosquito is a 1000 miles away according to Oxitech.

With all due diligence, I can only determine that our plan for the US is to rely on current surveillance and control techniques with a watchful eye out for where populations of Zika mosquitoes might appear and then attack with a vengeance. The problem with that plan is that by the time we discover such a pocket, more than a few of the mosquitoes have traveled onward or the virus is out in the population taking car rides a few hundred miles away to who knows where. If all of this sounds like so much finger crossing and dumb luck, I'd have to agree. I think we're merely pretending to have a plan and we're about to get punched in the mouth.

Your Plan

For most of us, any encounter with the Zika virus is going to be a nonevent, one where even if we are infected we'll know nothing of its happening. For about 1 out of 4 or 5 of us, it will be an experience similar to a long, mild flu with a rash, some achiness or pink eye. Of that 20-25% who have signs and symptoms, there will be about a quadruple chance by conservative current estimates that they experience the paralytic terror of Guillain-Barre syndrome, about the same odds apply to young women in the first trimester of pregnancy that their fetus will have its neural tube fold interrupted and the fetus suffer from microcephaly.

But odds are a funny thing. They can be manipulated. If you jump out of an airplane from 3,000 feet the odds are nearly 100% you'll bounce once and be dead. However, with the right equipment and some training on do's and don'ts, the odds reverse to near 100% you'll have the time of your life.

One item in our favor is that many of us in the US aren't all that outdoorsy, even preferring to spend time inside with a good view when we travel to our glorious national parks where we see most everything either from inside the car or out the picture windows of rustic lodges. We do the same at home by opening up windows that are screened to keep the bugs out, often times venturing outside to another screened in area like a gazebo or three season porch. But, eventually, we are outside and the chances of exposure to *A. aegypti* or *A. albopictus* are present.

There are two things to keep in mind. One is that both types of Zika carriers are daytime mosquitoes and the other is that they prefer urban-type environments over the countryside. The reason for the urban preference is that both mosquitoes are quite happy to do their breeding in any sort of container that is holding water, be it your bird bath, neglected rain gutter, that flower pot catch pan or hole in the top of a wooden post. Out on the streets where trash like cups or any other water holding item is not picked up for days or weeks, that'll do as well for a laying mosquito.

There is no vaccine for Zika as of yet, though a couple of companies are making noise that current vaccine manufacturing methods should be able to do the job. However, even if they have one in the lab at this moment, getting it into mass production first has to pass inspection for safety and efficacy, a time consuming process that may easily add a year. Thus, the earliest vaccine is possibly 2017. Scratch off vaccine as part of your plan.

Your plan is basic and simple and employs what the American Mosquito Control Association (www.mosquito.org) calls the Three D's—Drain, Defend and Dress. They have put up an excellent website with all sorts of mosquito information that is accessible and informative.   Following is what www.mosquito.org recommends what homeowners should do:

1. Rid the area of anything that can hold water--cans, tires, buckets, kiddie swimming pools or any other

containers that allow standing water. Empty flowerpot catches, cemetery urns or vases and pet dishes every 2 days.

2. Clean rain gutters and put up gutter screens that have window type screening. Large holed screens still allow for tree seeds to get in as well as mosquitoes. Additionally, well placed quality gutter screens keep you off the ladder. Check for standing water under or around structures or flat roofs. Inspect outdoor faucets areas and air conditioners for spill catches. Fix the drips and prevent puddles that may be present for several days.

3. Birdbaths and wading pools must be emptied once a week. Ornamental pools should have their water changed out or populated with minnows called mosquito fish. Decorative pools may be treated with biorational larvicides like Bti or S-methoprene containing products under limited circumstances. Commercial products like "Mosquito Dunks" and "Mosquito Bits" contain *Bti* and can be found at hardware or garden stores for homeowner use. Wellmark International sells Pre-Strike Mosquito Torpedo that kills developing mosquitoes using an insect growth regulator.

4. Empty low areas that collect water with drain tiles or by filling them in with dirt. Fill tree holes and stumps with mortars or spray foam sold in cans. Sometimes you can drill a drain hole to alleviate pooling water. Application of a *Bti* or methoprene will also work.

5. Check your septic system's drain field and make certain no standing water is allowed. Check animal water tanks and drain at least twice a week.

6. Check for trapped water in tarps used to protect equipment. Peak the tarp to drain off water.

7. Inspect for proper grading around foundations, driveways and gardens to ensure proper runoff.

8. Avoid excess watering. Puddling is a sign of too much water.

9. Report standing water in ditches and other public commons to a mosquito control or public health office. Attempting to rectify such a matter on your own could land you in hot water with the powers that be. Besides, they would like to know so as to understand the extent of any surveillance or vector control they may need to carry out.

10. Screen your windows. Cut down tall vegetation that gives resting spots for mosquitoes. Mow your yard regularly and apply a product listing synthetic pyrethroids like deltamethrin and lambda-cyhalothrin.

11. Dress in light colored clothes, long sleeves and pants. Avoid strenuous activity that causes you to sweat. Avoid using perfumes and scented soaps. Avoid using open footwear like sandals. There are mosquito repellant clothing lines with Permethrin you may want to consider that is sold through sporting goods stores and online.

12. If you spend time outside, you may want to use an insect repellent containing DEET, Picardin or Oil of Lemon Eucalyptus. Follow the directions and avoid the eyes, mouth or open wounds. Spraying on to your clothes is not recommended as it may stain them. Confine spray to healthy skin. The back of a person's neck, forearms and lower legs are target spots. Wash sprayed areas when no longer needed. Remember that more is not better. If the spray is dripping off of you, lighten up.
("American Mosquito Control Association-Control")[44]

Regards your own health:

*If you notice you have flu like symptoms such as rash, pink eye, joint pain or fatigue, see a doctor as soon as possible, keeping in mind that the testing window for Zika is short, 2-7 days.

*Keep abreast of your local news or check your local government websites for announcements on findings regards mosquito borne diseases. Use this information to take more diligent precautions.

* Women of child bearing age who are pregnant or sexually active should be extra careful. Dress defensively in long sleeves and light colored clothing. Use a repellant sparingly if you suspect you are pregnant or trying to become pregnant. If you find yourself in a high risk area for Zika, use birth control to avoid an unintended pregnancy. If you are in a high risk area, you may want to consider postponing pregnancy.

*If you suspect you are pregnant and in a high risk area, defend yourself using mosquito repellants, proper clothing, mosquito net for your bed and staying indoors. Establish a prenatal care provider and report promptly any flu like symptoms, joint pain, conjunctivitis (pink eye) or unusual fatigue so you can be tested for Zika.

* Keep in mind that microcephaly is generally not detectable until 16 weeks at the earliest and in some cases not until the third trimester or even until after birth. North Dakota, and very soon possibly Indiana, restrict abortions based on the reason of fetal defect no matter what week in the pregnancy. Also, many states restrict abortion after 20 weeks except under various circumstances such as to save

the life of the mother. The following website provides detailed information of state by state abortion restrictions: http://www.guttmacher.org/statecenter/spibs/spib_OAL. pdf

* If you are immunocompromised in some manner, extra diligence should be practiced in areas of known Zika outbreak. At this time, though, there is little known in the way of how Zika may impact such people as those compromised by HIV or other medical conditions other than extrapolating from other mosquito borne diseases such as dengue, yellow fever, malaria or chikungunya.

Afterword

(Grim News)

I have emphasized throughout the rapidly changing nature of the Zika epidemic. The latest word comes from the *New England Journal* Medicine where 72 women in Brazil tested positive for Zika and were followed. Ultrasounds found major birth defects in 21 (29%) of the fetuses. Even worse, it appears that Zika can trigger birth defects later than just the first trimester, possibly even into the third trimester. (Brasil, "New England Journal of Medicine", 2016)[45] The 29% figure is in line with my back of the envelope figures, underlining that I was avoiding hyperbole. The latest study has more than enough grim news for those who tend to favor righteous plagues.

As of this updated printing, the situation regards the 2015-16 Zika epidemic in Latin America is still highly fluid regards the precision and breadth of knowledge of how the virus works and what are the true risks. There is enough well documented history to show that when we have trouble defining certain epidemics, that our lack knowledge is used as a mantle of false security. The HIV epidemic of the late 1970's and early 1980's is one epidemic where it was observed that gay men appeared sensitive to what was colloquially referred to as 'gay disease', 'gay plague' or 'gay cancer'. Not until 1984 was it discovered that the human immunodeficiency virus, HIV, was responsible for AIDS.

The initial reaction was bewilderment and no one could say for certain that AIDS was transmitted by sexual contact. Many didn't care and some even celebrated that the disease appeared confined largely to gay men. Researchers fought for funds to study the confounding and growing epidemic but more than a few political foes waged war against releasing any money, even private funds, for a disease they viewed as an act of divine justice against homosexuality. Not until it became strongly suspected that the disease was just as vicious and unrelenting in heterosexuals, and that it could be contacted by an infected needle stick or blood products transfusion, did the more recalcitrant powers of government relent to allow funding for research now that they understood the potential for harm.

As it stands in the United States, Zika is an other-world problem in places the vast majority of us will never go in countries many couldn't find on a map. While the World Health Organization and Pan America Health Organization have declared an international emergency, the call for action seems quite muted here in the United States despite fairly heavy media coverage. The Ebola epidemic totally inflamed the American public despite literally only a few fingers worth of cases within US borders. Making matters worse, Ebola carried mostly inaccurate images of massive hemorrhaging and certain, agonizing death with wildfire like contagion. The public reaction was a clamoring for draconian measures of quarantining entire countries and imprisonment of those who may have been in the presence of someone who was infected. In one instance in New Jersey, a perfectly healthy nurse who had been to West Africa where Ebola was on the march, was locked up in a tent in a hospital parking lot, a victim of political grandstanding by the governor needlessly feeding public hysteria.

Fortunately, there is no mass hysteria surrounding Zika here in the United States. Hopefully, this means cooler heads will continue to prevail in how we handle our first significant outbreak. However, the specter of several cases where some children come down with Guillain-Barre syndrome might be enough to trigger a massive over reaction that leads to things like cancelling outdoor youth activities such as soccer and baseball, shutting down outdoor pools and taking other outdoor related happenings off people's schedules. For Florida, a state that is defined by its outdoor tourist economy, they have reason to be nervous about a widespread Zika outbreak.

Yet, funding lags. Our now infamous do nothing Congress that has been infiltrated by an anti-science crowd that refuses to consider 1.9 billion in funding requested by the CDC for Zika efforts. As usual, President Obama has had to maneuver around a feckless Congress and managed to secure 585 million dollars originally budgeted for Ebola control, a robbing Peter to pay Paul scenario.

As of the first printing, 9 cases of US mothers have been identified as having the Zika virus. 3 of those mothers have delivered babies with two of those infants thus far appearing healthy(microcephaly sometimes does not reveal itself until later in the child's development) but the third has been diagnosed with microcephaly. Two other women miscarried but it is not known if Zika is the causing factor. Two women have had abortions with one doing so after fetal scans showed arrested brain development but there are no details on the second one. The remaining two women show no complications at this point.

Of those 9 we know with fair certainty two had pregnancies with a major cerebral birth defect, the two miscarriages are highly suspicious, four show no complications at this point and one we haven't enough information to make any health assessment. It would be fair to say that 4 of 9 are highly likely to have a Zika component. If such a ratio holds up as the virus spreads, we'll likely see more strident demands for more immediate and visible action.

Since the first printing and as of May, 2016, over 500 cases of Zika have been identified in the United States, excluding Puerto Rico. All have thus far been the result of the patients having travelled outside the country.

Meanwhile, Puerto Rico is suffering a 70 billion dollar debt crisis and Congress has had to intervene as of June 2016 to allow Puerto Rico to restructure its debt with its creditors. Of course, at such a point it means that Puerto Rico isn't exactly flush with funds to aggressively take on mosquito control efforts and as of May 2016 has several thousand cases with infections strongly suspected to be from their native mosquito population.

Complicating matters is that *A. Aegypti* and *A. albopictus* are both present in the Gulf Coast states plus Georgia and South Carolina with *A. aegypti* being the bigger culprit. The deep south states have higher rates of poverty and less window screens along with higher volumes of uncontrolled refuse along with perfect *A. aegypti* and *A. albopictus* habitat and climate. Further complicating matters for pregnant women is that Texas, Louisiana, Mississippi and Alabama prohibit abortion after 20 weeks unless the mother's physical health is endangered. Many women who are gestating a fetus with a major birth defect will have no definable specific threat to their own physical health thus in some states, by law, must carry the pregnancy to term. Florida prohibits abortion after 24 weeks except in cases of physical endangerment to the mother and Georgia at viability with the same exception as the other Gulf Coast states. The term 'viability' is a medically nebulous term when dealing with fetal birth defects since so many infants with major birth defects are viable but may need high risk surgeries or extraordinary care as they further develop. Texas's law is a mess in that they allow for abortion after 20 weeks if severe fetal 'anomalies' are discovered and defines 'anomaly' as 'incompatible with life outside the womb'. Darshak Sanghavi, a pediatric cardiologist, a fellow of the Brookings Institution and "Slate" health writer, illustrates the dilemma succinctly, writing, "*For example, defects resulting in long-term vegetative states,..... severe bodily deformities requiring repeated high-risk and painful procedures with an extremely low chance of success (massive congenital diaphragmatic hernias), genetic abnormalities causing death and severe disability but with a tiny chance of longer life (Patau syndrome) could theoretically not be "incompatible with life."* (Sanghavi, 2013)[46]

Who makes that call? Our court systems are notoriously bad for what is allowed as 'expert' testimony with egregious presentations of paranormal meanderings masquerading as science defended by known cranks and incompetents. Two such examples are handwriting analysis and bite mark analysis, both thoroughly discredited yet available for courtroom hire and used by prosecutors in many states. It has been discovered that drug sniffing dogs used in law enforcement are about as good as a coin flip at being correct about the presence of illicit drugs, yet the courts have ruled such drivel is still reasonable cause for a search even though the 'trained' dogs are so abysmally wrong. I cite these examples to call attention to the high likelihood that it is only a matter of time before some woman and/or her doctor will find themselves on the accused end of a prosecutor's legitimate or illegitimate expert claiming her abortion was a crime because the fetus would have been 'viable'. All this will be entirely dependent on the prosecutor's desires. Remember, the State needs only one crank no matter if every other expert in the field disagrees.

Since a major birth defect like microcephaly is only diagnosable late into a pregnancy, this puts the gestating mother in some states in a very real bind where she is pressed up against the 20 week deadline. At 20 weeks there very easily could be suspicion but not a firm confirmation of a major defect in the fetus. Once the mother crosses that line, barring a threat to her own physical health, she is legally obligated to carry the pregnancy to term no matter what is revealed in the following weeks. The other scenario is that a suspected major defect motivates the mother to terminate a wanted pregnancy where if she were not forced up against the 20 week deadline she may have taken her time to see for certain if she had a healthy fetus.

Then there is the issue of access to meaningful birth control to prevent unintended pregnancy altogether. As I mentioned in Chapter 8 *Matters of Conscience*, Texas counties that lost family planning clinics after funding was removed saw a 27% spike in pregnancies. Should this trend continue in states where our two threatening mosquitoes reside, there will an increased capacity for tragic outcomes. When we can't remove an organ for transplant from a deceased person without explicit consent from the deceased prior to their death or their legal surrogate, but can force a mother to carry to term a pregnancy where there is a major birth defect is confounding. The current political winds of women's' rights regards family planning meeting up with a Zika epidemic in the US is nothing except ominous.

Several Latin America countries are contemplating easing their abortion restrictions to allow termination of pregnancies where it is suspected that Zika may be contributing to microcephaly in the developing fetus. However, the heavy Catholicism that permeates Latino society is staunchly opposed to abortion. It will be interesting to see how it plays out but any nod towards women's rights is dubious.

Funding for mosquito vector control and surveillance here in the US shouldn't be too problematic but there are pockets of society who have already declared such funding is needless when all women need to do is not have sex to avoid a bad pregnancy. As of the third week of June 2016, Congress has been unable to agree on a Zika budget. The CDC asked for 1.9 billion dollars and several bills ranging from about 700 million to 1.1 billion dollars have made it the Senate floor only to fail to meet the required 60 votes due to the bills being bogged down with objectionable amendments such as, inexplicably, that the funding be cut from various federal birth control programs to offset the new spending. Some of the requested money was for mosquito control programs and coordination efforts. However, without that money, mosquito control districts and counties/states will be left on their own. Governor Scott and Senator Rubio of Florida have both expressed their exasperation over the foot dragging, a notable anecdote in that both are famous for opposing federal government spending on a range of health programs. Whether you may think it is just deserts such funding is being denied, it still leaves the 25 million citizens of Florida on their own to devise a plan.

There are 7 billion people on the planet Earth so someone is having sex and I don't expect it to stop anytime soon. Such an abstinence prescription is naïve and ignorant of the realities of human behavior and has zero business even being mentioned as plausible preventive measure to curb Zika pregnancies.

A magical vaccine is not on the horizon though there are glimmers of light, but they are too far off to help us this coming year. The best hope is to allow the mosquito experts to do their thing and make sure they have the funds to do so. Whatever objections there are to GMO mosquito releases need to be quelled with solid science to put the anxious at ease and not let misinformed hysteria remove what is probably the singularly most effective weapon we're going to have available to tamp down mosquito populations. After mosquito control there is our own personal action plan regards our homes and selves that will lessen the instances of transmission. The quote at the beginning of the book from Mike Tyson is entirely apt for what we are facing. As of now, the best chance we have is to have a plan and stick to it because we're about to get punched in the mouth.

Richard Mertens

Zika Facts

- In the world there are between 1175 to 3,000 known species of mosquitoes, depending on who is doing the classifying. The United States has 176 known species of mosquito.

- Only two types of mosquitoes within the United States are known to be capable of harboring and transmitting the Zika virus: Aedes aegypti and Aedes albopictus.

- Aedes aegypti is found in Texas, Louisiana, Mississippi, Alabama, Georgia, South Carolina and Florida with scattered pockets in the bordering states. Isolated populations have been documented in Arizona, New Mexico and California

- Aedes albopictus is found in Texas, Louisiana, Mississippi, Alabama, Georgia, Florida, South Carolina, Tennessee, Kentucky, Indiana, Illinois, North Carolina, Oklahoma, Kansas, Missouri, Virginia, West Virginia and Ohio. Small, isolated populations have been found in Wisconsin, Minnesota, Pennsylvania and New Jersey.

- Both A. aegypti and A. albopictus can propagate by laying eggs in water containers as small as a bottle cap.

- Both types of mosquitoes are aggressive daytime mosquitoes as opposed to most other types of mosquitoes that tend to be active in the early morning or late evening hours.

- The United States is currently an immunologically naïve population, meaning there isn't a widespread immunity to Zika since it is a new disease to the US, thus leaving all US citizens susceptible to an infection reaction.

- Zika is sexually transmittable and can stay present in male semen for up to 60 days. It may well be longer but as of May 2016 no testing beyond that has been done but is in progress.

- Condoms can lower the risk of transmission of sexually transmitted Zika though it is advised known infected males should abstain from sex especially in the presence of a partner who does not practice birth control.

- Zika is sexually transmittable via male on male sex.

- Zika affected babies do not always exhibit obvious maladies such as microcephaly. Zika affected babies can be born appearing normal only to have various conditions such as vision, hearing or other physical and mental delays or deficits appearing months later. Some infectious disease experts are quietly fearing a Zika caused issue may not appear for years and be manifested as immunological disorders or psychiatric disorders such as schizophrenia.

- 80% of people infected with Zika display no signs or symptoms.

- 20% of people infected will have mild fever, fatigue, aches and pains. In much rarer instances, Zika infection may cause the paralytic condition Guillain-Barre.

- It is not known definitively if Zika can be transmitted through saliva.
- Zika is not an airborne disease.
- A pregnant woman can be infected with Zika, display no signs or symptoms and still have a Zika affected baby. It is not known if women who do display signs and symptoms of a Zika infection have a higher risk for negatively affected pregnancies or if those who display no signs and symptoms have a lower risk of Zika affected pregnancies.
- The May 25, 2016 edition of the Washington Post reported, (I paraphrase): "Typically, microcephaly occurs in .02 percent to .12 of 1% percent of all U.S. births. By comparison, more common congenital conditions like Down syndrome is under 1 percent. The New England Journal of Medicine found the estimated risk for microcephaly with Zika infections in the first trimester of pregnancy ranged from 1 percent to 13 percent."(*Zika Virus and Birth Defects — Reviewing the Evidence for Causality*, May 19, 2016 Vol. 374 No. 20 authors S.A. Rasmussen, D.J. Jamieson, M.A. Honein, L.R. Petersen pp 1981-1987) NEJM
- There is no vaccine for Zika as of June 2016 though there are at least two promising vaccines in trial. The earliest would be mid to late 2017 should all things go well. As of June 2016, Congress has refused to authorize a budget to fight Zika.

Notes

Chpt 1 Notes

[1]Associated Press. *Voice of America.* August 3, 2015. http://www.voanews.com/content/ioc-to-test-rio-olympic-water-venues-for-viruses/2896440.html (accessed February 3, 2016).

[2]Jamaica, The Government of. *Ministry of Health, Government of Jamaica.* November 23, 2015. http://moh.gov.jm/epidemiological-alert-increase-of-microcephaly-in-the-northeast-of-brazil/ (accessed February 3, 2016).

[3] "Wikipedia." *Standard deviation.* Jan 27, 2016. ("Wikipedia "Standard deviation"", 2016, p. https://en.wikipedia.org/wiki/Standard_deviation) (accessed February 3, 2016).

[4]Pan American Health Organization/World Health Organization. "Epidemiological Alert:Increase of Microcephaly in the northeast of Brazil." PAHO/WHO. November 17, 2015. http://moh.gov.jm/wp-content/uploads/2015/11/2015-nov-17-cha-microcephaly-epi-alert.pdf (accessed February 3, 2016).

[5]Seattle Times. *The Seattle Times Nation & World.* January 26, 2016. http://www.seattletimes.com/nation-world/zika-virus-may-be-linked-to-surge-in-rare-syndrome-in-brazil/ (accessed Feb 4, 2016).

[6]Haroon Siddique, Matthew Weaver. *Mail & Guardian.* Feb 1, 2016. http://mg.co.za/article/2016-02-01-who-holds-emergency-meeting-on-zika-virus/ (accessed Feb 4, 2016).

Chpt 2 Notes

[7]Wikipedia. *Aedes albopictus.* Feb 4, 2016. https://en.wikipedia.org/wiki/Aedes_albopictus (accessed Feb 4, 2016).

[8]US Dept of Health and Human Services. *Centers for Disease Control and Prevention.* Feb 4, 2016. http://www.cdc.gov/chikungunya/resources/vector-control.html (accessed Feb 4, 2016).

[9]Devlin, Hannah. ""Sweat and blood why mosquitoes pick and choose between humans"." *The Times*, February 4, 2010: unknown.

Chpt 3 Notes

[10]CostHelper.com. *Costhelperhealth.* not noted not noted, 2015. http://health.costhelper.com/shingles-vaccine.html (accessed February 6, 2016).

[11]Washington Post. *To Your Health.* February 3, 2016. https://www.washingtonpost.com/news/to-your-health/wp/2016/02/02/dallas-reports-case-of-zika-spread-through-sexual-transmission/ (accessed February 6, 2016).

[12]Wall Street Journal. *World.* February 3, 2016. http://www.wsj.com/articles/brazil-identifies-two-cases-

of-zika-transmitted-by-blood-transfusions-1454544342 (accessed February 6, 2016).

[13] Washington Post. *To Your Health.* Feb 1, 2016. https://www.washingtonpost.com/news/to-your-health/wp/2016/02/01/zika-virus-who-declares-global-public-health-emergency-given-rapid-spread-in-americas/ (accessed Feb 6, 2016).

[14]Centers for Disease Control & Prevention. *Immunization Schedules.* Feb 1, 2016. http://www.cdc.gov/vaccines/schedules/easy-to-read/child-easyread.html (accessed Feb 7, 2016).

Chpt 4 Notes

[15]*Andre Strohl.* January 2, 2016. https://en.wikipedia.org/wiki/Andr%C3%A9_Strohl (accessed February 8, 2016).

[16] National Center for Biotechnology Information. Accessed February 09, 2016. http://www.ncbi.nlm.nih.gov/pubmedhealth/PMHT0024547/.

[17] Wikipedia. "Cytomegalo Virus" February 9, 2016 Accessed February 09, 2016. https://en.wikipedia.org/wiki/Human_cytomegalovircy.

[18] "Mycoplasma Pneumoniae." Wikipedia. November 15, 2015. Accessed February 09, 2016. https://en.wikipedia.org/wiki/Mycoplasma_pneumoniae .

[19] Wang, David J., David A. Boltz, Janet McElhaney,

Jonathan A. McCullers, Richard J. Webby, and Robert G. Webster. "No Evidence of a Link between Influenza Vaccines and Guillain-Barre Syndrome–associated Antiganglioside Antibodies." Influenza and Other Respiratory Viruses. September 29, 2011. Accessed February 10, 2016. http://www.ncbi.nlm.nih.gov/pmc/articles/PMC3595170/.

[20] "VAERS - Vaccine Adverse Event Reporting System." VAERS Data. Accessed February 10, 2016. https://vaers.hhs.gov/data/index.

Chpt 5 Notes

[21] "Data Table of Infant Head Circumference-for-age Charts." Centers for Disease Control and Prevention. 2001. Accessed February 11, 2016. http://www.cdc.gov/growthcharts/html_charts/hcageinf.htm.

[22] Purves, Dale. "Box D Brain Size and Intelligence." National Center for Biotechnology Information. Accessed February 11, 2016. http://www.ncbi.nlm.nih.gov/books/NBK11129/box/A1833/.

[23] "NINDS Anencephaly Information Page." Anencephaly Information Page: National Institute of Neurological Disorders and Stroke (NINDS). June 30, 2015. Accessed February 12, 2016. http://www.ninds.nih.gov/disorders/anencephaly/anencephaly.htm.

[24] "New Link between Zika Virus and Microcephaly Is

Found in Brazil." PBS. February 4, 2016. Accessed February 13, 2016.
http://www.pbs.org/newshour/updates/new-link-between-zika-virus-and-microcephaly-is-found-in-brazil/.

Chpt 6 Notes

[25] "Zika Virus and Plasma Protein Therapies." Plasma Protein Therapeutics Association. Accessed February 13, 2016.
https://www.haemophilia.ie/uploaded/files/Zikavirus PPTA Statement.pdf.
   PDF document linked from www.haemophilia.ie

[26] Bevins, Ent. "In Brazil, Carnival-goers Won't Let Zika or Economic Woes Ruin the Party." Los Angeles Times. February 6, 2016. Accessed February 15, 2016.
http://www.latimes.com/world/mexico-americas/la-fg-brazil-carnival-20160206-story.html.

[27] Riker, David, and Jessica Vila-Goulding. "The Boom in Brazilians Traveling to the United States." *Journal of International Commerce and Economics*, January 2013.
https://www.usitc.gov/journals/JICE_Boom_in_Brazilians_Traveling_to_US.pdf.

[28] Amesh A. Adalja, Tara Kirk Sell, Nidhi Bouri, and Franco. "Lessons Learned during Dengue Outbreaks in the United States, 2001–2011 - Volume 18, Number 4- April 2012 - Emerging Infectious Disease Journal - CDC." Emerging Infectious Disease Journal - CDC. March 15, 2012. Accessed February 15, 2016.
http://wwwnc.cdc.gov/eid/article/18/4/11-0968_article.

Chpt 7 Notes

[29] Schuler-Faccini, Lavinia, PhD, and Et Al. "Possible Association Between Zika Virus Infection and Microcephaly — Brazil, 2015." Centers for Disease Control and Prevention. 2016. Accessed February 17, 2016. http://www.cdc.gov/mmwr/volumes/65/wr/mm6503e2. htm?s_cid=mm6503e2_w.

[30] Racaniello, Vincent. "Zika Virus and Microcephaly." Zika Virus and Microcephaly. February 10, 2016. Accessed February 17, 2016. http://www.virology.ws/2016/02/10/zika-virus-and-microcephaly/.

[31] Podulka, Jennifer, M.P. Aff, Elizabeth Stranges, M.S., and Claudia Steiner, MD M.P.H. "Statistical Brief #110." Statistical Brief #110. April 2011. Accessed February 18, 2016. http://www.hcup-us.ahrq.gov/reports/statbriefs/sb110.jsp.

[32] "Mapping Health: Mapping Maternity Care and Birth Outcomes." Mapping Health: Mapping Maternity Care and Birth Outcomes. Accessed February 18, 2016. http://www.mappinghealth.com/maternitycare.

[33] "Giving Birth in Canada: The Costs." Giving Birth in Canada. Accessed February 18, 2016. https://secure.cihi.ca/free_products/Costs_Report_06_E ng.pdf.

[34] Stevenson, Amanda J., MA, and Et All. "Effect of Removal of Planned Parenthood from the Texas

Women's Health Program — NEJM." New England Journal of Medicine. Accessed February 20, 2016. http://www.nejm.org/doi/full/10.1056/NEJMsa1511902 #t=articleTop.

Chpt 8 Notes

[35] Kaplan, Sarah. "Texas Health Official out of Job over Study Favorable to Planned Parenthood." Washington Post. February 19, 2016. Accessed February 22, 2016. https://www.washingtonpost.com/news/morning-mix/wp/2016/02/19/texas-health-official-out-of-job-over-study-favorable-to-planned-parenthood/?hpid=hp_no-name_morning-mix-story-f-duplicate:homepage/story.

[36] GBD 2013 Mortality and Causes of Death Collaborators. "Global, Regional, and National Age-sex Specific All-cause and Cause-specific Mortality for 240 Causes of Death, 1990-2013: A Systematic Analysis for the Global Burden of Disease Study 2013." Lancet. December 18, 2014. Accessed February 22, 2016. https://www.ncbi.nlm.nih.gov/pmc/articles/PMC4340604/.

[37] "Abortion Statistics, Facts About Abortion In The US." Abortion Statistics, Facts About Abortion In The US. Accessed February 22, 2016. http://www.womenscenter.com/abortion_stats.html.

[38] "Unsafe Abortion." Wikipedia. December 12, 2015. Accessed February 22, 2016. https://en.wikipedia.org/wiki/Unsafe_abortion.

[39] Lewin, Tamar. "Ohio Bill Would Ban Abortion If Down Syndrome Is Reason." The New York Times. 2015. Accessed February 23, 2016. http://www.nytimes.com/2015/08/23/us/ohio-bill-would-ban-abortion-if-down-syndrome-is-reason.html?_r=0.

Chpt 9 Notes

[40] "Venezuela Doctors Fume as Health Ministry Fails to Publish Data on Zika Cases - Firstpost." Firstpost Venezuela Doctors Fume as Health Ministry Fails to Publish Data on Zika Cases Comments. 2016. Accessed February 24, 2016. http://www.firstpost.com/world/venezuela-doctors-fume-as-health-ministry-fails-to-publish-data-on-zika-cases-2601002.html.

[41] "Zika in Texas." – Health Care Professionals. Accessed February 24, 2016. http://www.texaszika.org/healthcareprof.htm.

[42] "Controlling Adult Mosquitoes." EPA. Accessed February 25, 2016. http://www.epa.gov/mosquitocontrol/controlling-adult-mosquitoes.

[43] Specter, Michael. "The Mosquito Solution - The New Yorker." The New Yorker. Accessed February 26, 2016. http://www.newyorker.com/magazine/2012/07/09/the-mosquito-solution.

Chpt 10 Notes

[44] "Control." American Mosquito Control Association-Control. Accessed February 27, 2016. http://www.mosquito.org/control.

Afterword Notes

[45] Brasil, Patricia, MD, and Et Al. "Zika Virus Infection in Pregnant Women in Rio De Janeiro - Preliminary Report — NEJM." New England Journal of Medicine. March 4, 2016.
http://www.nejm.org/doi/full/10.1056/NEJMoa1602412#t=articleResults.

[46] Sanghavi, Darshak. "Who Has an Abortion After 20 Weeks?" Slate. July 12, 2013. Accessed February 27, 2016.
http://www.slate.com/articles/health_and_science/medical_examiner/2013/07/texas_abortion_ban_after_20_weeks_prenatal_testing_reveals_birth_defects.html.

ABOUT THE AUTHOR

Richard Mertens' interest in writing about medical topics is an offshoot of his background as a registered nurse. He has experience with infectious disease outbreaks ranging from institutional seasonal influenza to nosocomials such as MRSA and clostridium difficile to the West Africa Ebola epidemic. His prior written work includes *"Ebola Safari: One Nurse's Experience Inside the Sierra Leone Epidemic"* published December, 2015.

Zika Virus: The Pregnancy Plague
©2016 Cerebral Issue Press
Cerebralissuepress.com
cerebralissuepress@outlook.com

Zika Virus: The Pregnancy Plague
©2016 Cerebral Issue Press
Cerebralissuepress.com
cerebralissuepress@outlook.com